FUNDAMENTAL BASIS OF
IRISDIAGNOSIS

THEODOR KRIEGE

FUNDAMENTAL BASIS OF IRISDIAGNOSIS

A concise textbook

Translated from the German by
A. W. PRIEST, F.N.I.M.H., M.B.N.O.A.

L. N. FOWLER & CO. LTD.
1201/1203 HIGH ROAD
CHADWELL HEATH
ROMFORD RM6 4DH
ESSEX

ISBN 085243 332 8

The Random House Group Limited supports The Forest Stewardship
Council (FSC®), the leading international forest certification organisation.
Our books carrying the FSC label are printed on FSC® certified paper.
FSC is the only forest certification scheme endorsed by the leading
environmental organisations, including Greenpeace. Our
paper procurement policy can be found at
www.randomhouse.co.uk/environment

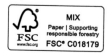

Printed and bound in Great Britain by Clays Ltd, St Ives PLC

CONTENTS

FOREWORD TO THE SECOND EDITION

When I published my books—*Disease-signs in the Iris*—several years ago, I then stated that these publications were not textbooks in the true sense of the term. Subsequently, I received so many enquiries for a concise textbook that I published the following work, of which the second edition now appears.

My main purpose has been to provide the serious beginner with an understanding of the basic concepts, so as to enable him the more easily to absorb the extensive material contained in the works of Dr. Schnabel, Angerer, Deck, Hense, Jensen and Maubach.

This second edition enables me to include the results of research and experience gained over the past few years.

It is my hope that further investigation will succeed in establishing a single uniform schema. Signs of this are already apparent.

THEODOR KRIEGE

Osnabrück, 1968

FOREWORD TO THE FIRST EDITION

When I published my books—*Disease-signs in the Iris*—some years ago, I had to point out that these small works were written strictly within the limits of the title. Consequently, many enquiries were received for a brief textbook of the fundamental principles of Iris-diagnosis.

Since the older original texts are now out of print, and difficult to obtain second hand, I therefore decided to publish the present work. The book will provide the beginner with a concise presentation of the material contained in the works of Dr. Schnabel, Angerer, Deck, Hense, Jensen and Maubach.

The basic iris-schema used conforms strictly to the system of Frau Eva Flink, and although this does not agree with other systems in all respects, yet the dissimilarities can be reconciled.

I hope that a later generation will succeed in establishing a single uniform system. In spite of zealous efforts, these have so far not succeeded.

THEODOR KRIEGE

Osnabrück, 1962

FOREWORD TO THE ENGLISH EDITION

The friendly reception which the first edition has found at home and abroad encourages me to issue the second edition. So much the more so since the opportunity is thus provided to include in the text the experience of more recent years.

It is due to the initiative of A. W. Priest, F.N.I.M.H., M.B.N.O.A., that this second edition appears in the English language, and I wish to express my thanks to him.

I hope that the edition will help to stimulate the exchange of knowledge and experience among iris investigators all over the world, as well as to provide a basic text for those interested. Only so can research into the subject become increasingly more profound and successful.

THEODOR KRIEGE
Member of the World Iridology
Fellowship

Osnabrück, 1968

A. First Part

Fundamental Basis of Irisdiagnosis

Chapter 1

The History of Irisdiagnosis

Before commencing the study of Irisdiagnosis, it is necessary to clarify two terms which are always being confused: Iris-diagnosis and Eye-diagnosis.

These two terms are not synonymous. Irisdiagnosis is the observation and diagnosis of disease from the iris, and is sometimes referred to as Iriscopy. Eye-diagnosis is the observation and diagnosis of diseases affecting the whole eye, including the pupil and iris, and the immediately surrounding parts. Strictly speaking, this should be referred to as Ophthalmoscopy.

The observation of changes on, in, and around the eyes is very old. References to it are found in the works of Hippocrates, as also in the Medical School of Salerno, and in Philostratus. The first reference to it by a physician of more recent times is found in the work of Philippus Meyens. In his book *Chiromatica medica*, published in Dresden in 1670, he draws attention to the signs in the iris and their interpretation. His comments on irisdiagnosis are here quoted for their historical significance:

. . . The upper part represents the head. Since the stomach has a close relationship to it, then all diseases originating in the stomach are found in the eyes. The right side of the eyes shows the state of all organs inside the body which lie on the right side, such as the liver, the right thorax and the blood vessels. The left side of the eyes can show all organs which lie on the left side, therefore the heart, left thorax, spleen and small blood vessels. Conditions of health and disease arising from the heart are found here, especially weakness of the heart or fainting. . . .

The lowest part of the eyes represents the genitalia and also kidneys and bowels, from which colic, jaundice, stone, diseases of the gall and venereal diseases are to be found. These signs consist of vessels, weals and flecks. If the eyes have far too many lines and flecks they signify a state of unhealth in respect of the whole body. Red lines or flecks signify hot-bloodedness. White flecks indicate watery blood. . . .

(Quoted from Herget aus Rossdorf)

Somewhat later the works of Johann Siegmund Eltzholtz appeared, in Nürnberg, 1695. In 1786, Christian Haertels published in Göttingen a dissertation under the title *De oculo et signo* (The eye and its signs).

Even though the significance of the eye was acknowledged in olden times, and special attention directed to it, nevertheless almost all these works refer even more to the Symptomatology. The complete examination, comprising inspection of the urine, diagnosis from the hand, nails and facies, assessment of hereditary taints, and diagnosis from the tongue, are neither taught nor acknowledged today in the technical colleges, with the exception of urine analysis where there is some acceptance. However, it is very important to remember that up to the beginning of the nineteenth century, such methods were an important part of orthodox medicine.

The true discoverer of Irisdiagnosis in its present form was the Hungarian physician—Dr. Ignatz von Peczely (1822–1911). In the year 1881 he published the method in his work—*Discoveries in the field of Natural Science and Medicine: Instruction in the study of Diagnosis from the Eye.*

On the basis of several decades of comparative study, von Peczely taught that certain indications in the iris were to be related to organic diseases, and that from the localisation of such a sign conclusions could be drawn as to the disease of the corresponding organ. He developed an iris-topography in which every organ had its proper place. According to Peczely's iris-chart of 1881, the right half of the body is projected into the right iris, and the left side of the body into the left iris.

The head and thorax are shown correspondingly in the upper half of the iris; the arms, abdominal organs and legs in the lower half of the iris. Medially placed organs are localised in both irides. The heart is shown in the left iris at 3 o'clock (15 mins). The whole area inside the iris-wreath is correlated with the gastro-intestinal tract, showing the ascending colon in the right iris, the transverse colon in both irides, and the descending colon (including sigmoid and ampulla) in the left iris.

(Quoted from Herget)

In the year 1893, the Swedish pastor Liljequist brought out a work entitled *Om Oegendiagnosen*. The book consisted of 284 pages, and an atlas with 258 monochrome and 12 coloured double-iris drawings. At first, he maintained that he developed eye-diagnosis independently from Peczely, and goes so far in the above work as to correct Peczely's statements.

From about the year 1887, the Tübingen ophthalmologist Schlegel supported Irisdiagnosis. His book, *The Eye-diagnosis of I. v. Peczely*, was well known at that time. The names of others who were prominent at the turn of the century should be mentioned: Stiegele, Rapp, Wirtz, Zoepperitz.

However, these well-known names are superseded in significance by that of Pastor Felke (1856–1926), to whom the credit belongs for complete originality in this field. His eye-diagnosis, upon which he himself unfortunately never wrote, has been expounded by A. Müller in a book, *The Eye-diagnosis based upon the principles of Pastor Felke*.

Even after his death, Felke influenced the development of Irisdiagnosis through his pupils, whose influence is still evident today. To this group belong H. Hense, as well as Frau Pastor Madaus and her daughter, Eva Flink, together with many other indirect pupils. Many of these pupils have in their turn acquired student groups.

Other well-known authors and investigators should here be mentioned: Maubach, Dr. Schnabel and Thiel; Anderschou in England; Collins, Kritzer and Jensen in the U.S.A.; Vannier in France. The list may be concluded with the names of Angerer, Baumhauer, Deck, Kronenberger, Struck, Dr. Unger and Dr. Wermuth.

Much is still to be done, and many pages have yet to be added to the history of Irisdiagnosis.

Chapter 2

The Divisions of the Iris

The Radial, Circular and Sectoral division of the Iris

In studying Irisdiagnosis, we need first to learn the topography, that is, the divisions of the iris.

Nearly every iris researcher has tried to evolve something special for himself, with the result that varying perceptions and interpretations are current. With goodwill, all might be reconciled.

These differences are inevitable, for one investigator had no academic training, and presented his observations in the language that was familiar to him, while others had already studied medicine and made use of scientific qualifications. Some considered the colour changes more (Liljequist), while others were chiefly concerned with the location of signs (Peczely). It should also not be forgotten that many signs may appear according to the locality, and in consequence of nutritional and climatic influences.

This book will endeavour to present the best, the most useful, and generally considered most important information from all systems. What is the most important?

If one wishes to commence something it is usual to make a plan, either on paper or at least in the head. We shall also do so. For the purpose, the iris is divided radially and circularly.

Radial division: The pupil is surrounded by a circular formation—the iris. We will begin with the radial division of this circle. (See Figure 1.)

The figure shows three possibilities—division of the iris into minutes, hours and degrees. The division into degrees 1–360 is too small for the purpose. The hourly division 1–12 is indeed familiar to everyone, but is rather crude for the precise location of iris signs, whereas the radial division into minutes 1–60 is suitable for all purposes. For those who wish to keep to the degree or hourly division it will suffice, but in this book, the 1–60 division will be followed.

Circular division: Now note the second most important aspect of iris topography, namely, the circular division. From the pupil to the outer border of the iris the area is divided by concentric rings. Each of these divisions is called a Zone.

In comparing the available literature in this respect we find considerable differences. Not only are many zones specified, but their names are very different. Peczely names three zones—a stomach, an intestine and an outer zone. He speaks, however, of regions. This division, with slight differences, is also given by Felke, Hense, Anderschou, Collins, Kronenberger, Baumhauer and Maubach. Vannier, Wirz and Kritzer specify only two regions. Schnabel mentions three zones. However, he names as the first zone the one he calls the 'Neurasthenic ring', as the second the stomach, and as the third the intestinal zone. Frau Pastor Madaus, Frau Eva Flink and Struck divide the iris into three large zones or six small regions—or as we would now say—zones. Dr. Bernard Jensen of California also names six regions, not including the pupillary margin. Thiel is a particular exception, he has specified several narrow and wide rings in his system. In connection with this, there are also various interpretations.

In this book the division of the iris according to Frau Eva Flink will be adopted, using the designation Zone. Passing to the consideration of the iris structure, we note immediately around the pupil a fine dark-to-light brown border which is quite narrow, and which we designate: Pupillary margin. The real objective of observation is the 'edge' around the pupil. The alternative term—Neurasthenic ring—was coined by Rudolph Schnabel. Colour changes and organic lesions of this ring indicate disturbances of the central nervous system.

The iris itself is divided into three major, or six minor equal zones. On examination of the iris a particularly striking change in the course of the iris fibres is noticed. This interruption in the course of the fibres, which normally includes about one-third of the iris, is called the Iris-wreath. On close examination we find this first one-third division, i.e. the first major zone, normally subdivided, and including the first and second minor zones. This part of the iris is also known as the pupillary zone. If the iris-wreath is not visible, then one has to reckon with pathological disturbances. (See Figure 2.)

The further division of the outer two-thirds of the iris, also called the ciliary zone, is less striking in terms of change in the iris fibres. However, this area is arbitrarily divided into two major, i.e. four minor equal zones. That it is important to examine the iris according to this division will be seen later from the study of the positions of the organ and disease signs.

This scheme of division was first introduced by Frau Pastor Madaus in her system. Frau Eva Flink and Colleague Struck also made use of the same schema. If we bear in mind the three major and six minor zones, as seen in a normal iris, there will be less likelihood of misinterpretation.

The *First Major Zone* contains the organs of food preparation and resorption:

First minor zone—stomach.

Second minor zone—intestines.

The *Second Major Zone* contains the organs of transport and utilisation, with elimination through the kidneys:

Third minor zone—blood and lymph vessels.

Fourth minor zone—muscular system.

In this zone we also have the positions for the organs: heart, kidneys, adrenals, pancreas and gall-bladder.

The *Third Major Zone* contains the organs for body support and ultimate utilisation, including detoxication and elimination:

Fifth minor zone—skeletal system.

Sixth minor zone—skin.

Detoxication: liver and spleen.

Elimination: through nose, mouth, urethra, anus and total skin.

Sectoral division (see Figure 3): Besides the division into zones, it is necessary to define the exact position of individual organs. For this purpose, the iris is divided into sections by drawing lines from the outer border to the pupil. Frau Madaus writes in her book on this method:

> The division of the iris into one-half, quarter, eighth, and sixteenth, including the 'change-over' and insertions, establishes the mathematical structure and harmonic relations of irisdiagnosis in general. Each division shows a front and back or sideview of the body. Furthermore, it establishes as lying diametrically opposite each other, that which naturally belongs and functions together.

In these words, the so-called 'change-over' is explained.

If a diagram of the iris is divided into four equal quadrants by a vertical line drawn from top to bottom, and a horizontal line drawn from right to left, as shown in Figure 3, the body divisions belonging together will not be under one another, but opposite each other.

Thus, in the iris, the areas for face and neck lie in the upper nasal quadrant, chest and abdomen in the lower temporal quadrant. Occiput and clavicle lie in the upper temporal, and the back in the lower nasal quadrant. In other words: by 'change-over' one understands that the front view of the body lies in the upper half of the iris nasalwards, and in the lower half of the iris temporalwards. Correspondingly, the posterior body lies in the upper half of the iris temporalwards (laterally) and in the lower half of the iris nasalwards (medially).

The above will have clarified the concept of 'change-over', so let us pass on to consider the above-mentioned dividing lines and their interpretation. (See Figure 4.)

Half and Quarter division of the Iris

1. The *Vertex-Foot line* = Equilibrium line—is an imaginary line erected through the middle of the iris from top to bottom, dividing the iris into an inner and outer segment (nasal and temporal segments: medial and lateral segments). Since the vertex lies in the upper part of the iris, and the foot in the lower part, it is named the Vertex-Foot line. If this imaginary line actually registers in the iris, through lightening or darkening, then the patient is subject to disturbances of equilibrium. Hence, it is also referred to as—Equilibrium line.

2. The *Throat-Neck line* = 'change-over' line—also called the Disharmony line—divides the iris into an upper and a lower half. It runs from the throat area in the iris which lies medially (nasalwards) in both irides, to the neck which lies laterally (temporalwards).

In the upper half of the iris lie all the organs of the head, besides the heart, lungs and other respiratory organs. In the lower half of the iris lie all organs which are between the neck and the feet. In the upper half of the iris we also have the special sense organs, larynx, trachea and oesophagus. In the lower half of the iris we have chest, back, abdomen, abdominal and pelvic viscera, and extremities.

When this Throat-Neck line registers, there exists a disharmony between the head and the rest of the body, hence the term: Disharmony line. Hyperthyroidism, coupled with heart and lung disturbance, is a possibility.

The Eightfold division of the Iris

3. The *Nose-Diaphragm line* takes its course through the middle of the upper medial quadrant and the lower lateral quadrant, from the root of the nose to the spleen area in the left iris, or to the liver area in the right iris. In the lateral segment it represents the boundary line

17

between chest and abdomen, which in the body is represented by the diaphragm. Hence, it is named the Nose-Diaphragm line. White lines traversing the right iris in this area suggest conditions terminating in violent pains. It is therefore also termed: Pain-line. Similar signs in the corresponding area of the left iris suggest terminal pains arising from febrile conditions. (Splenic enlargement = inner fever.)

4. The *Ear-Bladder line*, which is drawn through the middle of the upper lateral quadrant and the lower medial quadrant is interpreted as Infection-line. It commences above in the ear area, and traverses the bladder area below. If this line has a dark registration in the right iris, it suggests the existence in the antecedents of severe chronic bladder disease. As practitioners, we must ascertain in diseases of the ears in children, whether the ancestors had disease of the bladder. On this basis arises the right Ear-Bladder line, also called Hereditary-transmission line, because it reveals the connection with hereditary encumbrance. In the right iris the bladder sign appears when catarrh of the bladder follows chill. If signs are seen in the bladder area of the left iris, then we should mainly think of venereal disease.

The Sixteenfold division of the Iris

5. The *Mouth-Hand line*. If a line is now drawn midway between the nose and throat lines in the upper medial quadrant, continuing to the outer iris margin between the neck and diaphragm lines in the lower lateral quadrant, we produce a connection between the mouth area in the upper medial quadrant, and the hand area in the lower lateral quadrant. This line is called the Mouth-Hand line, also Nutrition line. Registrations in this location signify that the patient suffers nutritional defects. These patients will not change their eating habits. If this line shows in the right iris, it suggests that the ancestors suffered from diseases of the stomach. If in the left iris, then the patient has always eaten that which he is unable to digest.

6. The *Forehead-Ovary line*. If commencing with the forehead boundary in the upper medial quadrant, which lies midway between the Vertex and Nose lines, a line is projected to the margin of the lower lateral quadrant between the Foot and Diaphragm lines, we have the Forehead-Ovary line. Registration of the line indicates disturbance of sex life with effects upon the brain, in this case the emotional nature. Women with ovary signs and short stubby finger nails have much head pain, and also usually have many children.

7. The *Cerebellum-Uterus line/Cerebellum-Rectum line*. A line drawn

in the right iris from the margin between the Vertex and Ear lines, through the upper lateral quadrant, commences with the Cerebellum. In the lower medial quadrant the line runs midway between the Foot and Bladder lines to the area for uterus. If there are registrations of this line in the right iris, then the patients are noisy and incline to hysteria. Vertex headaches are then predominant.

In the left iris we have the Cerebellum-Rectum line, which as the name implies, does not run to the uterus area but to that for the rectum and anus. Registration of this line suggests conditions terminating in hypochondria. Such patients are quiet, and have little to say.

8. The *Axilla-Loin line*. This line is drawn midway between the Ear and Neck lines through the upper lateral quadrant. Here we have the area for axilla and clavicle. In the lower medial quadrant the line is drawn midway between the Bladder and Throat lines, and so demarcates the area for Loins. This line is the Axilla-Loin line, or Endurance line. Patients showing this line are very sensitive. One must not demand too much of such patients. They can neither bear nor endure much. (See Figure 4.)

Chapter 3

The Colour of the Iris and the Iris-layers

(See Figure 5)

The colour of the iris determines the appearance of the eyes. We distinguish in general three natural basic colours: blue, grey, and brown.

Each of these colours has a physiological basis, and is conditional upon the degree of pigmentation of the iris.

The iris appears blue when its surface layers are colourless, and the deepest dark layer of the iris (retinal epithelial pigment) shows through. If the middle vascular layer of the iris—the stroma—is coarse and compact, then the iris appears grey. However, the more dark coloured material is deposited in this stroma, the more the iris is darkened in its colouring, and the appearance tends towards brown. There are occasionally seen in a less pigmented iris, local accumulations of brown-to-black coloured substance which strikingly appear as dark-reddish flecks in the otherwise grey or blue iris. These are referred to scientifically as naevi irides (iris-birthmark). We call them 'toxin-flecks'.

In the case of albinos, the iris layers are completely transparent. There is a lack of all pigment. These eyes appear reddish, because of the visibility of the blood vessels in the deep layer of the iris—the retina.

In the new-born, the iris is at first dark-violet to blue-grey. Only in the course of development does there appear a lightening or darkening through alteration in the pigment content. With advancing age the stroma becomes more compact and coarser and thereby acquires a grey appearance.

The change of blue to brown iris is sometimes limited to an individual iris or even to a part, so that in the same person, one iris can be blue with the other brown, and also a smaller or larger brown sector may be seen in the blue iris. This is referred to as Heterochromia. Discolourations of the iris following organic diseases are of especial significance in Iriscopy. These discolourations will be considered later in Chapter 6.

The structure of the iris is best viewed when the pupil is contracted, using a strong beam of light, either with natural vision, or better still with a loupe of 3 or 4 magnifications.

The iris is rich in changes, and is especially characterised by elevations and depressions of the anterior surface. This is referred to as the iris-relief.

The Layers of the Iris

From anterior to posterior the iris is organised in the following layers:
1. Endothelial
2. Anterior marginal layer
3. Vascular layer = Stroma
4. Posterior marginal layer = Dilatator layer
5. Epithelial pigment = Stratum pigmenti iridis
6. Retinal layer = Pars iridica retinae
   (See Figure 5)

1. The question of the existence of the Endothelial layer is not completely settled. Many researchers assume an anterior membrane of the human iris, others dispute it.

2. The anterior marginal layer is composed predominantly of cells, between which lie numerous nerve endings but few blood vessels. Cells bearing colour material—Chromatophoren—may be present, which together with the stroma gives rise to certain colour changes in the iris. Where the marginal layer is missing, smaller or larger dark-shining openings—so-called crypts—tissue spaces, allow a view of the interior of the spongy iris—stroma. These crypts will be considered later as lacunae.

3. The Vascular layer, or iris-stroma, constitutes the principal bulk of the iris. It consists mainly of numerous blood vessels which radiate in spokes, and therefore run radially from the outer margin of the iris towards the pupil. The blood vessels are enveloped in a thick adventitia of connective tissue fibre, and are surrounded by a loose ramifying network and pigment cells, which fill out the spaces between the blood vessels.

These blood vessels appear as spiral formations below the anterior marginal layer. In these formations they can adapt to the conditions of expansion and contraction of the iris.

Besides the radiating blood vessels of the iris stroma, there is in the iris an arterial ring arising from the annular anastomosis of the ciliary blood vessels—the Circulus arteriosus iridis minor. It is situate at the border between the pupillary zone and the ciliary zone, and is called in Iridology the Iris-wreath.

In a very light iris one can also see a grey band at the pupillary margin. This is composed of smooth muscle fibres which surround the pupil in a ring-formation. They form the sphincter of the iris—Sphincter pupillae —which lies in the iris-stroma.

4. The posterior marginal layer—Dilatator layer—joins on to the posterior surface of the vascular layer. It consists of a continuous layer of spindle-shaped smooth muscle fibres, extending from the outer margin of the iris to the ciliary border near to the pupillary margin. Here it unites with the connective tissue of the sphincter.

5–6. The epithelial pigment forms the posterior surface of the iris and extends to the pupillary margin, around which it runs to the anterior surface of the iris, thereby giving rise to the frequently visible dark-yellow to black-brown pupillary margin.

This margin, where the fibres reflect back, is the only structure in the human body, which as the embryological representation of the central nervous system, provides a surface accessible to view.

This posterior pigment layer consists of two layers of epithelial cells which pass over into one another to the pupillary margin. (Stratum pigmenti iridis with Pars iridica.) Both together form the continuation of the retina as far as the pupillary margin. Thus, this layer of the iris is denoted Retinal, in contrast to the anterior layer which is called the Uveal. (Pars retinalis iridis, and Pars uvealis iridis.)

Apart from the structure referred to above, examination frequently reveals a number of light or dark concentric arc lines. These are seen particularly frequently in a brown iris where they stand out because of their light colour on a dark background. These are the 'contraction rings' of the iris, which in Iridoscopy have a special meaning.

Quite remarkable are the groups of white flakes seen at the periphery of the ciliary zone, and sometimes scattered regularly around the whole iris like a rosary. These will be discussed later under the heading 'Acute or chronic inflammation of the mucous membranes'.

At the periphery, there appears a partial, or frequently entire, dark almost black circle (Scurf rim). In old age it becomes obscured by a silver-grey rim projecting from the sclera (Sclerotic rim). The black circle is formed by the crypts of the ciliary margin, and the silver-grey rim results from fatty infiltration—it is a sign of senile change (Arcus senilis).

Chapter 4

How do the Iris-signs Originate?

In order to make a thorough investigation of the iris-signs, it is first necessary to consider which type of sign. We distinguish three kinds of signs in the iris:

1. Unnatural colourings.
2. White, dark and black signs—chiefly as dots, radiating lines or 'wisps'.
3. Circular signs—called 'Contraction rings'.

1. The unnatural colourings have their basis in the circulatory fluids of the body. These circulatory fluids (blood and lymph) are affected by external and internal influences, as through medication, or autointoxication, and changes due to uric acid or biliary disturbances. These pathological changes in the lymph are revealed not only by the skin and mucous membranes, but show also in the iris and the sclera, as is evident in jaundice. There are also the deposits in tissues, as may occur in rheumatism and gout.

For details of unnatural colourings, see Chapter 6.

2. Special attention is given to the white, dark and black signs of the iris which are generally radiating in direction, and which constitute the first consideration in the recognition of disease conditions. White signs may also indicate unnatural substances, as with uric-acid crystalline deposits, arteriosclerosis, etc.

The next signs to investigate are the inflammation-signs. These appear with acute diseases, and either disappear on recovery, or become darker and darker with the transition to the chronic phase, and ultimately change to black signs with the direct loss of tissue-substance in the organs concerned.

White signs mean: Over-stimulation, increased activity, heightened rhythm (e.g. peristaltic), and irritation of the nerve-fibres.
Dark signs mean: Insufficient stimulation, diminished activity,

23

atony, atrophy, loss of substance: the iris shows loss of colour, thus becoming darker, and with the final destruction of nerve fibres and tissue cells ultimately registers as black signs.

When there is destruction of the nerve-plexus of an organ, how is it that neither the connection nor the result is visible in the iris? It is functionless, and hence useless. In the same way, we can find a plausible explanation for the white healing-signs surrounding the black signs in the iris which indicate loss of substance. It suggests that there is increased functional activity in the tissues adjacent to the nerve plexus —exactly the same in the organ as in the iris. Either the healthy fibres assume the functions of the destroyed nerve pathways, or alternatively initiate a reparative activity by laying down new tissue (scar-tissue) and promoting fibrosis.

In the same way, one can explain the traumatic-lesion signs found in the iris—frequently showing a characteristic shape, i.e. according as whether caused by a blunt or pointed object. It then shows not the form of the instrument but the shape of the injury, as for example the destroyed tissue and nerve cells.

There are also the so-called 'lacunae'—small or large open spaces in the iris, which are more easily visible, the more plentiful their surroundings of interweaving thick vascular trunks. These (lacunae) lie between the delicate reticular ramifications of the nerve bundles and indicate functional weaknesses. The ramifications also suggest a weakened organism. The 'lacunae' usually appear in the iris in large numbers, if present at all.

3. **Contraction rings.** Circular signs, called Cramp rings (Nerve rings) which appear as shorter or longer segments of arc, are found only in the ciliary zone. These 'ring-furrows' are usually lighter or darker than the remainder of the iris and arise in connection with conditions of continued spasm. Considerable difference of opinion exists as to their origin.

Schnabel ascribes to a slackening or spasm of the sphincters or dilators of the ciliary muscles. Thiel believes that through the continuous regular pull of all the dilator fibres, or at least of a sector of the iris-diaphragm, functioning in the same way as the pupillary margin, that concentric arcs would be formed by circular folds.

Now it is surely remarkable that these rings are found only in the ciliary zone, usually in arcs of smaller or greater length, and this is highly suggestive when it is also observed that not more than four such arcs are to be found running parallel. Surely, it must be considered that the arc-shape makes it fairly improbable that the radiating fibres of the pupillary dilators could form these rings.

With close observation of the ciliary zone in the normal iris we find three concentric interruptions faintly signified. How do these arise? According to the opinion of Frau Pastor Madaus, they arise in the true nerve fibre. Dr. Andogsky states that these enter the iris in radial bundles. Thereafter they immediately lose their radial direction and turn parallel to the ciliary border, thus forming the first ring, and thereafter sending several thick radial branches towards the pupillary margin with a number of smaller branching distributions.

After which, the larger nerve branches which have traversed approximately a third of the distance to the midway of the total width, again turn parallel to the border and conjoin to form arcs—the second ring. From these, radiating branches project to form a new line of arcs close to the iris-wreath: the third ring. We thus have three concentric contracting rings of iris nerves.

If we apply our understanding of the origin of the white and black radial signs to the nerve rings, then it follows that their bright or dark appearance must be related to conditions of over-stimulation or deficient stimulation. The arc formation of which the individual rings consist readily explains the appearance of partial rings. If we find a region of the body as localised in the iris so marked, we may certainly assume that these rings give definite indication of disturbance in such parts.

Whether such are always associated with painful attacks—spasms— I cannot confirm, since one frequently finds that there is no history of such conditions. From my observations it appears that cramp-like conditions exist in the bodily organs corresponding to the iris region where the nerve rings show an interruption.

In dealing with 'nerve-rings' we must also consider the zone in which they are found. If registering in the Blood-zone, then they indicate disturbances of circulation in the large blood vessels and lymph channels. If found in the other zones—muscular, skeletal, skin— then disturbances exist in those tissues.

During the last twenty years, the incidence of these nerve rings has increased ten to fifteen times. I attribute this to the calcium deficiency arising from the bad nutrition of the war years.

Chapter 5

The Iris and the Constitution

I, myself, agree with the views of Pastor Baumhauer of Vienna on this subject. Since I am in accord with him, I quote here from his statements literally:

> The increased research of hereditary factors will enable Iriscopy, as well as the constitution of an individual, to be determined in the widest sense. By constitution, one understands the total of inherited and acquired factors, which determine the actual quality of the blood and lymph, and which in turn result in the state of the remaining bodily organs and tissues. In short: the entire constitutional condition of a man in his ability to withstand the disease producing influences. A constitution reflects the genotype insofar as it is qualified by hereditary factors. Beyond that, it may be modified within certain limits by environmental influences occurring during the course of life (domestic circumstances, nutrition, social factors).
>
> However, it must be stipulated that it is not disease as such but only the dispositions which are transmitted, and that, moreover, from the very first moment of intra-uterine life an effective influence is required to precipitate the actual disease. The total of these tendencies and influences provides the complete picture of the constitution of man (phenotype).

The most valuable aspect of Iriscopy lies in the ability to make a rapid estimation of the human constitutional disposition by an examination of the colour and structure of the iris. The colour of eyes, hair and skin is collectively referred to as the complexion, and these three generally remain in close relation to each other. Since this complexion derives from the blood and other body fluids, certain inferences may be drawn regarding the composition of the blood as well as the morphological structure of the whole organism. The constitution is thus comprehended in terms of chemical and biological functions. Let us take the ground colour of the iris as the principal criterion for the classification of constitution. We thus obtain three main groups:

    i. Blue iris—blond hair, fair skin
    ii. Grey iris—mixed and compound forms
    iii. Brown iris—dark hair, dark skin

It is obviously possible to draw finer differences, such as the lighter and darker shades within all three colourings, but these will here be disregarded. Let us now attempt, in a general way, to give the characteristics of the three different constitutions.

Blue iris: The blue iris is the expression of thinner blood. We have here nothing less than the lymphatic constitution known of old. Von Paltauf has written:

> Enlargement of tonsils, lymph nodes, extended lymph node complex of the follicles at the base of the tongue, enlargement of the spleen and the presence of an abnormally large thymus gland at a time when this should have quite disappeared.

Their origin lies in the lymphatic constitution of childhood, during which the lymphatic system and the lymph are already in a condition of hyperfunction. Arising from a continuance of this lymphatic constitution throughout childhood, certain lymphatic and torpid conditions develop during growth and puberty, of which the main examples are: adenoidal growths, nasal polypi, enlarged tonsils, swollen lymphatic cervical glands, swelling of the thyroid gland, and transitional states developing Basedows syndrome and exophthalmic goitre. These are the typical characteristics of this iris colour.

This type has a particularly distinct predisposition with regard to the respiratory system: asthenic pulmonary states, pleuritic and bronchitic conditions, haemoptysis and tuberculosis, here produce most victims. There is also a greater tendency to reabsorption of uric acid with greater accumulation in blood and body fluids, giving rise to rheumatic and neuralgic disturbances. Arteriosclerosis and corneal opacity is more frequent with this type. Heart and kidneys are found to be more easily susceptible.

To summarise: the following are the typical characteristics—blue iris, lymphatic-rheumatic-tubercular constitution.

Grey Iris: The grey iris, which is due to the reinforcement of the connective tissue fibres of the vascular layer, has a constitutional similarity with the blue iris, but with a special tendency to rheumatic-catarrhal affections involving septic skin conditions such as acne, furunculosis, obstinate skin eruptions; and as a secondary consequence of suppressed perspiration strong catarrhal secretions from all the mucous membranes.

As a result of insufficiency of the renal secretions with noticeably disturbed conditions of quality and quantity of the urine, there arise many unrecognised and difficult conditions of disease of obscure origin.

Summarising: The grey iris is the sign of a rheumatic-catarrhal constitution.

Brown Iris: The brown iris results from a larger concentration of pigment cells, and suggests above all a greater concentration of blood and body fluids.

An admixture of a greater or smaller quantity of bile pigment frequently lends the eye a greenish shimmering lustre. Because of the concentration of blood, and arising from various environmental and domestic influences, the deficient digestion of this type is a character-istic feature with a special predisposition to diseases of the digestive system, of the gastro-intestinal canal along with the associated organs: gastric atony, nervous dyspepsia, constipation, with their secondary states of flatulence, stomach pains, and gastric and duodenal ulcers. These unfavourable tendencies more frequently appear in the female sex with the following consequents—cephalalgia (headaches), choleli-thiasis, appendicitis, abdominal plethora (abdominal stasis—particularly of the portal system) and signs of congestion, as well as neurasthenia (sensitive nervous weakness) and hysteria (also psychoneurosis).

The functional tendencies consist of a morbid sensitivity of the liver, so that slight disturbances of bile secretion arise from dietetic errors, such as jaundice, hepatic eclampsia, and inflammation of the gall-bladder. Concentrated and cholesterin-rich blood may also aggravate any tendency to new growths.

To summarise: Brown iris—gastric-bilious-carcinomatous constitu-tion.

Thus, by observing the basic iris colour, one may determine in every human being the relatively weak aspect of his organism which is in the slightest degree susceptible to disease-producing influences, and which therefore merits particular consideration from the outset.

It by no means always requires a complicated and exhaustive clinical examination, but merely Iriscopy in conjunction with the history, sex, age and occupation, in order to establish the constitution with its particular predispositions, and thereby to determine quite easily in what respects it has a prophylactic significance.

Apart from the colour of the irisis, there is also the actual structure, with its special indications of a constitutional deterioration in the resistance of the total organism, and a decrease in general vitality. Of particular significance is the integrity of the anterior (superficial) layer of the iris as revealed by the greater or lesser degree of delicacy and strength, and through which it is possible to see the underlying supportive connective tissues and vascular layer. This integrity is an indication of the resistance factor in the total organism.

Disregarding the colour of the iris, and assessing only the integrity of the anterior superficial layer we have the following:

1. *Ideal Iris:* a fine textured iris with an unbroken surface, without crypts or contraction rings (nerve rings).
2. *First-grade Iris:* an iris texture with little trophic change affecting the anterior layer, although small crypts are evident, especially in the area of the iris-wreath. People with such an iris are in general extremely resistant of constitution, and mostly enjoy untroubled health.
3. *Normal Iris:* partial atrophic change of the anterior layer, revealing larger portions of the deeper vascular layer, a greater prominence of the iris-wreath, and disproportionate distribution of pigment.
4. *Degenerative Iris:* almost complete atrophy of the anterior layer, honeycomb-like network of the connective tissues of the vascular sheath, a star-shaped distortion of the iris-wreath, and considerable infiltration of the chromatophors in the deeper layers of the stroma, indicating a deep degeneration of the vital state, and at the same time suggesting the detrimental effects upon the organism of hereditary influences.

The difficult question of the connection of the constitution with a definite mento-emotional habitus can merely be referred to here. The influence of the soma upon the psyche and the reverse is firmly established, as well as the supremacy of the mind over everything material. A satisfactory explanation for it is given only by the theory of psycho-physical correlation in human nature, in which body and soul, although essentially different from one another, are yet naturally co-ordinated in combinations which constitute human substance.

Chapter 6

Interpretation of Iris-signs

Iris signs, from which a disease state can be diagnosed, are differentiated

    (*a*) By their colour
    (*b*) By their shape

A. Colour of Iris Signs

The colouring of iris signs has already been explained in Chapter 4, 'How do the Iris-signs Originate?' It was stated there that white, dark and black signs can appear:

1. *White signs* are signs of inflammation or over-stimulation. The whiter the signs, the more acute, inflammatory and painful is the condition of the affected organ. If the condition becomes chronic, then the originally white sign changes to blue-white, dirty-white, yellow or even brown.

The white iris signs show only in blue and grey irides as so brightly white. In brown eyes, the acute state shows only as a lightening of the brown iris tissues, which are then brighter than the background shade, but never quite white.

2. *Dark iris signs* are signs of under-stimulation, diminished function, and enervation. The iris shows in the appropriate region—grey to dark grey, but yet not black. These signs are always to be seen where the superficial surface layer of the iris has receded to expose the second layer—vascular layer (= the lacunae and dark wispy signs).

The dark iris-signs denote a chronic disease state of the tissues as suggested above in referring to the yellow to brown signs. The difference between these two groups is to be found in the cause of the actual disease conditions. Those described under 1. above are signs resulting from the deposition of toxic wastes and residues in the tissues. They are indications of a state of tissue which has been described by N. Krack in *Erfahrungsheilkunde 5—1961* as follows:

These signs are symptoms of incomplete products of intermediate metabolism which infiltrate into the interstitial connective tissue and there induce degenerative processes, indurations and loss of fluid. This process is progressive, attacks always the connective tissues, and can even encroach upon vascular and nerve fibres.
[This quotation does not originally refer to iris-signs—T. Kriege.]

As against the signs just described, which originate from an excess in the tissues, and which become visible in the iris as deposits, are those described under 2. above: dark iris-signs indicating over-relaxed tissues with tendency to tissue destruction and consequent atrophy.

3. *Black iris signs* indicate loss of substance. They originate from the destruction of the second layer of the iris, which thus allows the third pigment layer to become exposed.

4. *Coloured signs in the iris*—also called toxin-flecks—can appear as yellowish-red, rust-red, brown, black-brown, or in all other shades. They lie mainly in the deeper iris-layers. These foreign colourings will be explained later on in this book, but it may here be noted that Dr. Schnabel in his book *Iridoskopie* has written fully on these different forms and colours. Angerer also treats these indications fully in his work, *Handbuch der Augendiagnostik*.

B. Form of Iris-signs

The shape of iris-signs varies considerably, and in the early stages of study easily produces difficulties of interpretation. I will here attempt to write fully and exhaustively on the description of each type.

1. *Lines:* One has to differentiate white and dark lines; short, long and zigzag lines. Short white lines are usually found lying in contiguity one with another, and are signs of inflammation affecting the organs concerned. Long white lines are those which are not limited to one organ area, but run over several areas. They are indications of neuritis with pain, or of neuralgia. They begin in the iris-wreath, or even at the pupillary margin, and run towards the outer border. If these lines run in zigzag fashion (see iris illus. 5 and 12), the patient will be found to complain of cramp-like pains. Such a zigzag line in the heart area is the sign of a cardiac neurosis (or irritable heart = D.A.H.). The patient will complain of the occurrence at times of severe palpitations. If one finds in the point of a zigzag line small black dots, then a danger of paralysis of the affected organ is indicated. (Nerve paralysis.)

Dark lines in an organ area are indications of nervous weakness.

31

2. *Flakes and Clouds:* These are always white to yellow-white. They appear as signs of an acute or chronic inflammation of the mucuous membranes (catarrh). The signs are usually seen in the form of small flakes directly around the pupil (inflammation of the gastric mucous membranes), or in the form of larger flakes or clouds in the mucous membrane zone (Minor zone 5), in the sectors for lungs, thorax, peritoneum, frontal sinus, etc. (See iris illus. 3, 6 and 8.)

3. *Wisps:* can be white, yellowish or dark. They are larger than clouds and flakes, and not so intensely indicated. They take in the entire organ area (e.g. as in uterine catarrh), or an entire zone (e.g. the muscle zone in general muscular rheumatism). White wisps are signs of an extensive tissue-inflammation. (See iris illus. 6, 7 and 8.)

Dark wisps appear when the indicated organ has become weak in reaction (often observed in the area for uterus). White wisps become yellowish in the transition to the chronic state, and in the course of time even brown. They appear as brownish or brown depositions in the superficial iris layer, and largely conceal the true basic colour of the iris. There are irides which are almost completely covered with this brownish deposit, and patients with such irides are persons who incline to stiffness and gout. In such cases the predisposition is hereditary, but these brown deposits are also to be seen as such in acquired conditions.

4. *Lacunae:* signs of weakness. Lacunae appear wherever the iris fibres diverge in small or large arcs and thus expose the second darker iris layer. They are indications of organic weakness. One must differentiate:

    (*a*) *Open lacunae*—when the iris fibres do not again converge towards the outer iris rim and join up. These signs signify that the defect is still in the early stages, not yet closed, and that therapeutics have yet to influence it.

    (*b*) *Closed lacunae*, when the iris fibres reunite towards the outer rim of the iris, thus forming an oval sign. A closed lacuna is the sign of a completed disease process. Closed lacunae may be acquired, as well as inherited. (See iris illus. 4, 5, 8 and 9.)

There are many variously shaped lacunae, which all have a special meaning. Angerer and Schnabel have written on them in great detail.

5. *Honeycomb signs:* are lacunae in which small white lines provide a honeycomb appearance by running lengthwise and across within the lacunae. (See iris illus. 2.) These indications suggest contraction of the organ (atrophy), with hardening and scar-tissue formation.

6. *Black dots:* and also oblong or jagged small black lines, suggest

tissue-disintegration, loss of substance, ulcers. Where ulcers are healed, a fine white line surrounds the black sign—the so-called healing ring.

7. *Transverse signs:* or 'adhesion' signs, are very fine white lines which run obliquely across the iris structures. They are also referred to as 'cobweb' signs. They are indications of adhesions and agglutinations, and are often found in the pleural area and in the caecal area. If the transverse signs are covered with a small white cloud, then an acute inflammation is indicated, and the patient complains of pain. (See iris illus. 1, 4, 6 and 10.)

8. *Radii Solaris:* are radiating furrows in the iris tissues which are wider at the base and taper towards the outer rim. They can commence either at the pupillary margin or at the iris-wreath, and radiate towards the scurf rim. If one is seen in the brain area, then as pointed out by Angerer, a cerebral weakness is indicated. If appearing somewhere in the remaining iris area, it indicates that the organ in which sector it appears is affected by nerve weakness.

9. *Wedge signs:* are small black signs which are directed with their bases towards the iris-wreath. If such a sign is seen in the heart area, then the possibility of sudden death occurring must be considered. If appearing in the kidney areas, then a condition of contracted kidneys is indicated.

10. *Contraction rings* (Nerve rings)—earlier called 'Cramp-rings'—are concentric interruptions of the iris fibres which are especially seen in the second and third major zones. Three or four of these rings are often to be seen lying next to one another. They indicate circulatory disturbances in the tissue, and disturbance of lime metabolism. Interruptions in the continuity of the nerve ring indicate cramp-like pains in the organ sector concerned (gall-bladder, uterus, heart, legs, etc.).

With these contraction rings one must also consider the zone in which they appear. If they lie in the blood zone, then there will be disturbances in the large blood and lymph vessels. If they lie in the bone and skin zones, then one must expect to find disturbances in these organ systems.

11. *Local dilatations and contractions* of the iris-wreath and the intestinal zone. Contraction of the iris-wreath towards the pupil signifies a pressure or compression from outside affecting the intestine, e.g. from a tumour or swollen or displaced organ. Dilatation of the iris-wreath in round arcs, suggests a flabby state of the intestines. Pointed and jagged dilatations suggest colicky pains. (See iris illus. 1, 2, 3, 4, 9, 11 and 12.)

12. *Dark skin zone:* indicates a suppressed excretion. A milky-white scurf rim (arcus senilis) is a sign of arteriosclerosis. (See iris illus. 5.)

13. *Signs of death:* imminent:

    (*a*) A black wedge-sign in the heart area

    (*b*) Completely solid black scurf rim

    (*c*) A perpendicular-oval pupil

14. Besides the iris signs described, one must also consider whether the iris rim displays a normal circular form. In severe organic diseases the iris rim is flattened in the appropriate organ area. Pupillary deformations are also of great diagnostic importance. I would here refer to the very informative work of Schnabel: *Ophthalmo-Symptomatology.*

Chapter 7

Interpretation of the Topography of the Organs in the Three Major Zones (Six Minor Zones)

1st Major Zone—Stomach and Intestinal Zone (see Figure 6)

In considering the topography of the organs we commence with the first minor zone—the stomach zone. The stomach zone has already been indicated as the first zone in the circular division of the iris (see Plate 2). It is now necessary to identify the parts of the stomach in the right and left iris.

If the body is divided down the middle by a perpendicular line we have: Pylorus with about one-third of the stomach in the right half of the body. Cardia and two-thirds of the stomach in the left half of the body.

All organs on the right side have their place in the right iris, and all organs on the left side have their place in the left iris, thus:

Pylorus and one-third of the stomach in the right iris. The remaining two-thirds with cardia in the left iris.

By dividing the stomach horizontally through the middle we obtain an upper and a lower part for each iris. Considering the right upper part of the stomach, this will include an anterior and posterior view of the upper part of the pylorus with the right side of the lesser curvature. Since we have in both upper and lower halves of the iris a representation of the anterior, posterior and lateral views, we may determine precisely the different regions of the stomach from the iris. Similarly, we place the right lower part of the stomach in the right iris, and both upper and lower left regions of the stomach correspondingly in the left iris.

From Figure 6 we note that the pylorus is exactly in the middle, lying between the upper and lower halves of the right iris. Thus:

Upper half pylorus—Right iris nasal side—12′–15′—antero-lateral aspect.

—Right iris temporal side—45′–48′—posterolateral aspect.

Lower half pylorus—Right iris temporal—42′–45′—anterolateral aspect.

—Right iris nasal—15′–18′—posterolateral aspect.

The cardia, lying in the left side of the body, is represented only in the upper half of the left iris, at:

Left iris nasal—45′–50′—antero-lateral aspect.

Left iris temporal—10′–15′—postero-lateral aspect.

In my view we cannot place the cardia in the lower half of the left iris.

The second small zone is designated the Intestinal zone, which includes the duodenum, small intestine, and the large intestine with sigmoid flexure. We shall again require to identify the regions of the right side intestine in the right iris, to show right upper and lower intestine with anterior, posterior and lateral views. (See Figure 7.)

Of especial interest to us here is the duodenum. Since this, and that part of the stomach lying in the right side of the body is more frequently affected, there must be reserved to this area a large part of the iris. We find on considering the indications that the proximal part of the duodenum lies over the pylorus.

For this part of the duodenum we have shown in the iris the area 10′–15′ and 45′–50′ in the upper half, corresponding to the anterior, posterior and lateral aspects. The part of the duodenum which lies below the pylorus is seen in the lower half of the iris from 15′–20′ and 40′–45′.

The junction of the duodenum with the small intestine lies in the left half of the body, so the area for it is found in the lower half of the left iris from 40′–45′. That part of the small intestine lying in the right half of the body is found in the right iris from 5′–35′ with an intermediate position for a part of the duodenum. (See Figure 7.)

At 35′ in the right iris, the ascending colon commences with the caecum, and extends to 50′, allowing for the insertion of a part of the duodenum. Here the right flexure indicates the commencement of the transverse colon which extends to 5′. Where there is a diseased appendix (it possesses much lymphatic tissue as is well known) the signs are to be seen outside the intestinal zone at 35′.

In the left iris, the area for small intestine extends from 35′–55′, with inclusion of that part of the duodenum which lies on the left side of the body—as already referred to above under Duodenum.

The transverse and descending colon is to be found in the area 55′–25′. The sigmoid and rectum then extend from 25′–35′. The last part of the rectum with ampulla and anus lies at 32′–34′ in the muscle, bone and skin zones.

2nd Major Zone—Iris-wreath, Blood and Muscle Zones

In order to elucidate the second major zone—Blood and Muscle zone—it will be necessary to clarify understanding of the iris-wreath (= Autonomic wreath). As is well known, the nutritional substances absorbed in the stomach and intestines are not all taken up from the blood, but also partly from the lymph stream. Therefore, the state of the lymph stream as denoted by the iris-wreath must also be considered.

If the area for central nervous system is located directly around the pupil (Pupillary margin—Neurasthenic ring) then the area for the vegetative nervous system is to be located in the iris-wreath. The signs which appear in connection with disturbances of these systems will be described under the Sign-indications. (See Figure 10.)

The designation Blood Zone for the third minor zone is so chosen since the blood supports all organs of the whole body. Also, the continuous movement of the lymph occurs because of the pulsation of the blood and the effect of muscular activity upon the autonomic nervous system. As we realise, the heart must occupy a special position in this zone, and in fact the right heart is located in the right iris at 45′–50′, and the left heart in the left iris at 10′–15′. The aorta is located in the left iris at 8′–10′.

Besides the heart, the pancreas, kidneys, adrenals and hypophysis, are also located in the second major zone, with their particular signs commencing at the iris-wreath. (See Figure 10.)

The pancreas is seen in several places. The position of this gland in the body corresponds to:

The head of the pancreas—from 49′–52′ and 10′–12′ in the right iris. (The head of the pancreas is embryologically separate and extends to the transverse part of the pancreas.)

The long body and tail-end extends to the spleen, and is indicated when affected at 38′–42′ and 19′–22′, in both irides, also commencing directly at the iris-wreath.

The kidneys are shown when diseased at 28′–30′ in the right iris, and at 30′–32′ in the left iris. Like the kidneys, the suprarenal glands have their positions directly at the iris-wreath—in the right iris at 30′–32′ and in the left iris at 28′–30′.

The hypophysis lies, beginning close to the iris-wreath, in the right iris from 60′–63′, and in the left iris from 57′–60′.

37

The urinary bladder is also to be seen in the second major zone, at 23' in the right iris, and at 37' in the left iris. The prostate gland is sometimes shown at the same location adjacent to it, towards the iris-rim.

The gall-bladder has its area in the right iris from 37'–39', and the uterus from 26'–27'—also in the right iris. The area for rectum is found in the corresponding area of the left iris—32'–34'.

The tonsils lie at 13'–14' in the right iris, and at 46'–47' in the left iris. The disease signs of these last named organs, like the urinary bladder, prostate gland, gall-bladder, uterus, anus and tonsils, have no direct connection with the iris-wreath. One can thus distinguish between a gall-bladder and a pancreatic condition when presented.

The bronchi show their signs mainly as extending from the iris-wreath to the sixth minor zone (Scurf rim): right iris 43'–45', and left iris 15'–18'. The trachea registers in the right iris at 12'–14', whereas in the left iris the oesophagus shows at 46'–48' in the corresponding position.

The course of the great arteries and veins is indicated in Figure 8. In this diagram the muscle zone is also shown. In this case it is not a question of seeing all muscles, as for example those of the stomach and intestines, but of assessing the general state of the voluntary muscles and the heart muscle.

The state of the muscular system is shown in the iris by the appearance of the lacunae. If the lacunae appear inside the iris-wreath, then the state of the muscle layers of stomach and intestines is indicated. When small lacunae are observed outside the rim of the iris-wreath, then a lability of the circulation is indicated. When the lacunae extend to the muscle zone, then the muscle fibres of the organs indicated by the particular areas involved are weakened through defective blood supply. If the lacunae extend fully to the iris margin, then it indicates that even the bones and mucous membranes suffer from nutritional disturbances.

The different types of lacunae have been discussed in greater detail in Chapter 6.

3rd Major Zone—Bones and Skin

The third major zone is also divided into two zones—the fifth and sixth minor zones. The fifth minor zone is called the Skeletal zone. The position of individual bones and groups of bones is shown in Figure 9. Further iris research may eventually require many minor modifications to this schema.

When a condition of the skeletal system is presented the sign should never begin in the iris-wreath. It may project well into the muscle zone, just as it may also extend into the sixth zone—the skin zone. It is, however, a sign which is always localised precisely in the middle of the ciliary zone. On the other hand, a heart sign, for example is always found conjoined to the iris-wreath, as also are the pancreas, kidney and adrenal signs. But the leg area never begins in the iris-wreath. These facts should be especially noted.

The junction of the fifth and sixth zones—bones/skin—refers to the whole of the mucous membranes. This large and important organ system is found for the most part within the skeletal system, as for example with the pleura in the thorax, and the peritoneum in the abdomen. Therefore the condition of this system is to be seen in the iris at the junction of the fifth and sixth minor zones. There are also special signs which appear in affections of the mucous membranes. (For details see Chapter 6.)

In the sixth minor zone, the degree of skin activity can be seen. All body openings also have their places in this zone. The position of these organs is shown in Figure 10.

However, I would like to draw attention to the position in this zone of a few particularly important organs. The liver is placed in the right iris between 37' and 40' at the outer margin of the iris. In the left iris the spleen occupies a corresponding position—from 20'-23'.

The thyroid gland may also be mentioned—at 14'-17' in the right iris, and 43'-46' in the left iris. The cerebellum is indicated when disturbed or diseased in the right iris at 54'-56' and in the left iris at 4'-6'.

The lung areas extend from the blood zone to the skin zone and are shown in the right iris from 45'-50' and in the left iris from 10'-15'. (See Figure 10.)

Disease Signs of the Organs

Chapter 8

Diseases of the Gastro-intestinal Tract

Stomach and intestines have their iris positions in the first major zone, directly around the pupil. In contrast to the other organs they are concentrically arranged, and take in a third of the iris.

When looking at an iris, attention is first directed to the stomach and intestinal zones. In health the stomach and intestinal zones are of equal size. They take in a third of the iris and do not differ in essential colour and structure from each other. This normal form of the first major zone is very seldom found in these days. Let us therefore consider the disease signs:

A. Stomach zone

1. *Hyperacidity:* The stomach zone is lighter than its surroundings, almost white and elevated. The patient complains of heartburn. If the stomach zone is circular and with a sharply marked outer circumference, then there is swelling and cramp of the stomach. Such patients have a constant sense of pressure in the stomach with cramp, associated with eructations. (See iris illus. 1.)

2. *Gastric insufficiency:* The stomach zone becomes dark grey and sinks inwardly. There may appear black lines deeply furrowed in the stomach area, in which case there will be functional deficiency of the mucous membrane. These patients also complain of heartburn, which is in this case a false indication of acidity (= lactic acid). If with these signs the stomach zone is too small, then that is a sign of induration/sclerosis.

3. *Inflammation of the mucous membranes = Gastritis:* In this condition one finds small white flakes lying directly against the pupillary margin, especially when viewed with side floodlighting.

4. *Inflammation of the stomach muscle layer:* This is of a rheumatic nature, and shows small white flakes or clouds in the outer rim of the stomach zone (therefore on the boundary with the intestinal zone). Patients with these signs cannot tolerate cold food or drink—they have the feeling of 'a cold lump in the stomach'.

5. *Gastric ulcer:* (Ulcus ventriculi et duodeni). The ulcer shows itself in the stomach zone as a black point, and is most frequently found in the posterior wall of the stomach (right iris about 20′, left iris about 40′), and in the pylorus. In the pyloric area the signs are more oblong than round, and usually extend over into the intestinal zone (ulcus duodeni). An open ulcer is a black point or line which is accompanied by a small white cloud (black point or line = loss of substance, white cloud = tissue inflammation, therefore the pain). When the ulcer has healed, the black spot becomes surrounded by a fine white closed ring (healing ring).

6. *Gastric carcinoma:* Cancer signs are small putty-like steel-grey signs which shine out from the depths of the iris. The iris appears putty-like and 'smudged'. Not infrequently a stomach cancer develops, especially a scirrhous cancer, from the so-called Ulcus callosum. This is shown in the iris in the form of several serrated black spots which overlap each other. The iris is then seen to be flattened in the outer rim.

7. *'Nervous' stomach:* A red-brown stomach zone points to a toxic poisoning of the gastric nerves (= the so-called 'nervous' stomach). In most cases this colour change also extends over to the intestinal zone. Often also, radiations extend over the brain areas—an indication that any headaches have their origin in the stomach.

8. *Dropped-stomach = Gastroptosis:* When through over-contraction of the pylorus the muscle layer of the stomach weakens (= dilatation of the stomach), or when through general slackening of the abdominal muscles there arises a ptosis of the stomach, then this condition will be recognised in the iris by an expansion of the stomach zone—from 30′–45′ in the right iris, and from 15′–30′ in the left iris. If the stomach zone areas—right iris 45′–60′, left iris 60′–15′—are enlarged, then that is a sign of gastric enlargement/dilatation. The reason for this is the accumulation of gas in the stomach.

One also finds patients with an enlarged stomach zone—from 15′–30′ in the right iris, or from 30′–45′ in the left iris. Here it is the posterior wall of the stomach which is relaxed and which gives rise to the ptosis. (See iris illus. 2, displacement of the stomach zone.)

B. Intestinal zone

Disturbances of the intestines are recognised in the course and colour of the iris-wreath.

1. Dilatations of the iris-wreath are often seen. If roundish, they suggest an intestinal atony, and these usually stem from incompletely

cleared catarrhs of childhood. Dark spots in the dilatations are indications that the intestinal glands are no longer functioning. Patients with these signs had many colicky pains as children, with a history of always wanting to drink cold water (= intestinal scrofula).

If the signs are more honeycomb-like, then one speaks of 'wormnests'. That is to say, that the patients have suffered from worms. If worms are suspected, then other signs are searched for: undue activity of the pupils, dark rings under the eyes, signs of worms on the tongue, in the nose, and itching of the anus, etc.

Pointed white spokes of the iris-wreath which take in the second large zone are signs of intestinal colic.

2. A white iris-wreath is an indication for inflammation of the intestines. This inflammation often extends over into the lymph channels, to the fifth minor zone (mucous membrane zone). One can then observe thick radiating white lines from the wreath to the fifth minor zone, in which white clouds or flakes also appear. (See iris illus. 6, 7, 8.)

3. A contraction of the iris-wreath arises because of pressure from the outside, and can be caused by organ displacement (e.g. floating kidney, enlarged liver) or by a tumour. A downward depression of the wreath is a sign of ptosis of stomach or intestines. (See iris illus. 2 and 4.)

4. An expansion of the large intestine field in the direction of the heart area (left iris 10'–15', right iris 45'–50') enables one to diagnose 'Roemheld'. (See iris illus. 9 and 12.)

5. Tumour and cancer signs were described in the previous chapter.

6. All iris signs which originate from the pupil and traverse the iris-wreath indicate a participation of the central nervous system in the disturbed condition.

7. If in the left iris one finds an iris-wreath with a pointed serrated margin, a sign of weakness in the heart area, and an adrenal sign, then a vegetative dystony is indicated. The patient is full of inner disturbances, with troubles here and there, without it being possible to define a clinical condition. (See iris illus. 4.)

8. A square-shaped wreath always indicates a grave and incurable condition. Pancreas signs are always then to be found. (See Chapter 10 and iris illus. 3.)

9. The appendix area lies in the right iris—from 33'–35', directly at the wreath. In inflammatory states there shows a white sign = acute condition, or a yellow sign = chronic condition. One often observes in

this area signs of adhesions, which go out from the intestine and reach to the peritoneum. They arise after chronic inflammations, as well as after badly healed appendicectomies, and can produce considerable disturbance.

A black spike in the caecal area signifies that the caecum has become functionally incapable and shrivelled. Black or dark lines which go over or under in an arc, indicate displacement of the caecum. Very often it becomes adherent to the gall-bladder, peritoneum, ovary, Fallopian tube, etc.

10. Strong dilatations of the intestinal zone from 25´–30´ in the left iris and from 30´–35´ in the right iris, enable one to recognise the tendency to hernia. The iris-wreath is broken through at the point where the rupture ensues. If pain also appears, then white clouds in this area will point to an inflammatory state.

Small lacunae inside the iris-wreath indicate a disturbance in the gastro-intestinal secretions, arising from atony of the stomach and intestine musculature.

11. Special attention should be directed to the S. Romanum (Sigmoid flexure) and to the rectum. In many cases, the area for rectum, left iris 32´–34´, shows a white discharge-sign, as an indication of mucous membrane catarrh. Often, the iris fibres in this area separate from one another, and indicate a sign of commencing weakness (= atonic constipation).

Signs for haemorrhoids are seen in this area in the form of small dark spots. Apart from this, one not infrequently observes a very dark brown neurasthenic ring, and indications of stasis in the liver area, as symptoms of a portal congestion. With haemorrhoids, one usually finds very wrinkled eyelids. Interrogation reveals that these patients must often rub their eyes because they feel as if there were sand in them. A later indication of haemorrhoids is the presence of a red fleck in the lower eyelid. The more this fleck lies temporalwards, then the more analwards lie the haemorrhoids. The more it lies nasalwards, then the higher they lie. (See iris illus. 4.)

Chapter 9

Diseases of the Liver and Gall-bladder

The liver, the largest detoxicating organ in the body, has its place at 37′–40′ in the sixth minor zone of the right iris. The gall-bladder, which is both anatomically and physiologically connected to the liver, has its place at approximately 39′ in the fourth minor zone, and in any case in the right iris only.

1. Liver-disturbances

Inflammatory states of the liver register as white or yellowish clouds or wisps in the specified area. In the inflamed state, the liver is swollen as the result of congestion, which is indicated by the displacement of the iris-wreath towards the pupil, and also by the inwardly depressed nerve rings if these exist. At the same location may be seen the small arteries of the sclera, which when apparent, always indicate the existence of an inflammatory disturbance of the organ in the area to which they run. (See iris illus. 3.)

Where there are inflammation signs in the liver area, one must very carefully consider whether the white signs (clouds or wisps) are present only in the liver area, or whether they are merely part of the total sign commencing at the iris-wreath and extending over the gall ducts to the liver area. (See iris illus. 3.) In the first case the disorder concerns the liver only, and is due to a disturbance of the detoxicating function of the liver which becomes charged with blood from the organism. In the second case the disturbance arises from a disorder of the duodenum (usually ulcerated), and because of the extending inflammation, leads to gall stasis and inflammation of the gall ducts and liver. Here, therapeutics must first be directed to the duodenal disorder. (See iris illus. 8.)

Where there are inflammatory processes affecting the liver, and hence a lighter colour in the liver area, there will also be seen signs in the area for spleen—left iris 20′. With such liver disturbances the patient complains of severe flatulence, and signs for this will be seen in the intestinal zone.

Much more often, the sign of inflammation is seen as a darkening of the liver area, and this indicates diminished liver function, leading to more or less severe metabolic disturbances. With this sign, there is usually found a very dark neurasthenic ring, as an indication of portal congestion.

Small dark spots in the liver area are signs of sclerosis, and enable one to diagnose a commencing hepatic cirrhosis. The greater is the darkening of the liver area, the greater is the disturbance of liver function.

2. Disturbances of Gall-bladder and Gall ducts

1. The inflammatory gall-bladder disturbances are recognised by a lightening of colour in the gall-bladder area—white lines or wisps. It is usually a question of an inflammation extending from the intestine, as already stated in connection with inflammatory states of the liver, going out from the duodenum, and extending in proportion to the disturbance as far as the liver. Usually only white lines are seen = pain lines. (See iris illus. 8.)

2. Gallstones themselves do not, of course, register in the iris. However, their presence can be presumed when small dark spots are seen in the gall-bladder area. Gallstones lead readily to inflammation and to gall stasis. (Compare Chapter 13, Kidney stones.)

3. Fine white, generally serrated, lines indicate the tendency to colic. The same tendency is also indicated by nerve rings which interrupt in the gall-bladder and gall duct areas.

4. Not infrequently, one finds the gall-bladder and liver areas displaced in profile to about 41′–42′. Patients who have this sign are tainted by hereditary disease. Among their antecedents there must have been alcoholism. We must also remember here that diseases which show the organ signs displaced in profile, are either not healed at all or only with great difficulty.

Chapter 10

Disturbances of the Pancreas

Disease signs of the pancreas are found in both irides, corresponding to the position of the gland in the body, in both left and right at 20' and 40'. However, with extensive disturbance of the whole gland, signs even appear as well at 10' and 50' in the right iris.

As has already been noted in relation to stomach and intestinal diseases, there is a squaring of the first major zone, indicating an involvement of the total vegetative nervous system. It is then a question of a condition which is difficult to cure (see iris illus. 3, Sympathetic quadrant, after Dr. Schlegel). The following is to be noted:

(a) The pancreas has its indications almost at the four corners of this 'Sympathetic-quadrant'.

(b) This means that in the presence of the pancreas sign and the square shaped wreath, we have an incurable condition.

(c) Such corners are virtually the storm-centre in the iris in all disturbances of the digestive system.

(d) Pancreatic disturbances which relate to the glandular secretory functions of the organ show mainly in the right iris.

(e) The signs always commence at the iris-wreath and show:

i. As weakness signs with decrease in the size of the organ = trophic weakness.

ii. As lightening with inflammation = over-stimulation. With inflammatory conditions and the consequent increased blood supply and enlargement of the organ, there would be an inward depression of the iris-wreath.

iii. As darkening = signs of hypofunction, in the form of dark wisps, clouds or spots. In this case we usually find the tendency to a square-shaped wreath, and must regard the pancreatic insufficiency as a consequence of chronic gastro-intestinal disturbances, especially where there are indications

49

in the adjacent intestinal area. Often there will be found partly healed ulcerated conditions, which vary from scar-tissue to complete adhesions, particularly in the areas for pylorus, duodenum, gall duct and pancreatic duct, and which must be considered as cause for the pancreatic weakness.

With cancerous processes affecting the pancreas—usually the head of the gland, we find the dark jagged sign especially extending from 20', 40' right iris, but also appearing at 50' right iris. Since the liver is always associated with cancerous changes as the principal organ of metabolic exchange and detoxication, we find a darkened, blurred liver area as well as a flattening of the iris rim in this same area.

It is important to make an exact examination of the pancreas area in the left iris at 20'. A weakness sign there, or a darkening of the area, indicates that there is a hereditary disposition to diabetes. (See iris illus. 4.) If diabetes already exists, then the liver and kidney areas will show signs of encumbrance. Of course, the urine must then be examined for presence of sugar, and the patients interrogated for the presence of subjective symptoms of this illness.

As already mentioned in an earlier chapter, disease signs indicated in profile are always an expression of a grave condition. That goes especially for pancreatic disturbances, since this organ always shows its signs in profile.

Chapter 11

Diseases of the Heart and Blood Circulation

The Heart

Heart signs are seen in the second major zone: Blood and Muscle zone—locally at left iris: 10'–15', right iris: 45'–50'—commencing directly at the iris-wreath.

With heart signs, as with the entire iris, a lightening of colour signifies over-activity = inflammation, and darkening indicates under-activity = weakness.

With all cardiac conditions, more so than with other organ signs, one has to consider the entire iris, and in particular the blood zone, brain, liver, lung and kidney areas. In addition, the finger-nails, legs and lips should be examined, since these often give early indications.

Heart signs for individual conditions are:

1. *Endocarditis* (inflammation of the endocardium): shows small white flakes in the heart area, or short white lines, especially close to the iris-wreath in the blood zone.

2. *Myocarditis* (inflammation of the heart muscle): is recognised by the appearance of small white flakes or clouds in the muscle zone: in the middle of the heart area, or further outwards towards the skeletal zone. These signs are very often apparent during the course of, or following an infectious disease, and must then be regarded as very grave indications. These signs are also frequently to be found with so-called 'rheumatic' patients. With such people the whole iris is too white, and these patients complain of generalised rheumatic pains, e.g. in shoulder, neck, back muscles, etc.

With such patients one often observes merely a thick, white zigzag line in the heart area which shows a small white flake at its termination in the mucous membrane zone. In such cases it will be found that the patients suffer severely from changes in the weather, and complain of great uneasiness and anxiety from stormy weather.

3. *Pericarditis* (inflammation of the pericardium): the pericardium registers approximately at left iris: 15′–17′, showing clouds in the lower margin of the heart signs when there is pericarditis. Since pericardial disease very easily gives rise to adhesions, one should always give careful attention to the fine white adhesion-signs (transversals) in this area, as well as to the adjacent pleural area below.

4. *Cardiac neuroses:* are widely spread in these times of increased tensions, haste and anxiety. Since in many cases of neurotic disturbance no clinical evidence can be found, iris-diagnosis becomes an especially important help.

In the early stages, nervous disturbances of the heart are shown by a very fine white line which runs out over the heart area from the iris-wreath, roughly horizontally. The patients complain of disturbance and sudden palpitations (the heart beats 'up into the throat'). If this white line takes on a more acutely zigzag form, then stronger disturbances are probable. Patients with such signs usually have enlarged 'moons' on the finger-nails.

If near these fine white lines contraction rings are observed (i.e. nerve rings), which interrupt at the heart area, then there is a risk of cardiac spasm, resulting in the appearance of praecordial anginal attacks.

If the nervous heart disturbances have existed for some time, then the fine white lines become darker, i.e. grey to black; usually there is only a dark line to be seen, known as 'irritation line'. Patients with such signs have constant heart disturbance as a result of irritation, grief or fear. If the lines become somewhat wider apart and give rise to lacunae, then the patient will complain of an anxiety state. If these signs lie at about 10′–12′ (left iris) then according to Frau Flink there is a condition of heart oppression and dyspnoea; if they lie at 16′–17′ then agitation and excitement will give the patient the feeling as if the heart was being strangled. Patients with these signs have nail 'moons' which are too small, or are wholly or partly missing.

5. *Cardiac myasthenia* (heart muscle weakness): is shown by a darkening of the heart area, appearing as dark wisps, clouds, and closed or open weakness-signs. The iris fibres no longer run radially, but more or less in arc form. For so long as the dark signs are small (narrow) and the fibres only slightly separated, then the condition is one of simple debility of the heart muscle, but if not treated this becomes a heart

muscle weakness. The weakness-sign itself is usually evidenced above or below (also above and below) by a light well-defined arc. Frau Flink interpreted a well-defined upper arc as a tendency to asthmatic symptoms, which arise on slight exertion. In the case of a lower arc, then according to Frau Flink the patient can eat only little.

When in addition to these signs the stomach and intestinal zones are coloured brown, then every excitement affects the stomach of such a patient.

The wider the separation of the fibres in the muscles zone of the heart area, the greater the tendency to cardiac dilatation. If the weakness-signs are closed, then according to Frau Flink, the condition should be regarded as one of cardiac dilatation and cardiac weakness. Such patients must always be treated as for a heart condition, especially with feverish infections—e.g. rheumatic and renal conditions. If the weakness sign is not closed, but is open as far as the iris margin, then the condition is one of hypertrophy (Frau Flink). If besides the weakness-sign in the heart area one finds an overgrowth of the nail-quick on the fingers, then the patient suffers cardiac anxiety and oppression. In children this is a sign of fearfulness.

As is well known, a heart muscle weakness leads to stasis in the systemic and pulmonary circulation. With left cardiac insufficiency this gives rise to dyspnoea with cough and catarrh, whereas with right cardiac insufficiency there is liver and portal stasis, haemorrhoids and hydropericardium. Thus, with weakness-signs in the heart area, one always pays attention to the lung areas. Stasis here makes the lung fields appear dark, the patient complaining of cough and dyspnoea, especially at night. Cardiac asthma and pulmonary oedema are possible dangers.

In proportion to the extent of cardiac weakness, stasis signs may be found in the areas for liver and kidneys, together with a dark neurasthenic-ring, haemorrhoidal signs in the rectum area, and stasis signs in the extremity areas. These areas become dark and the iris fibres separate. (See iris illus. 5, Signs for oedema of the lower extremities.)

Small lacunae in the heart area are sometimes found even in small children, in which case the cause is attributable to the mother. If during pregnancy the mother suffered much irritation and worry then the child is liable to have a heart-area lacuna. Such children are very nervous, and remain affected throughout the whole of life.

6. *Cardiac valve lesions:* show in the iris as small black points in the heart area in the vicinity of the iris-wreath, lying in the upper part of this area. There may be one to three black points. The appearance of a

fourth point is a presage of death. Struck wrote on this matter in *Iris-Korrespondenz* as follows:

> a visible fourth heart point renders hopeless any measures to counter impending death. This iris indication is diagnostic of the last stages of struggling man.

Another sign in the heart area which is difficult to interpret is the black wedge-sign. It lies in the blood zone with its base to the iris-wreath and the apex pointing into the muscle zone. It indicates that the patient may suffer a sudden cardiac arrest.

If in the heart area one or more black points are observed in the blood zone (indicating valvular defects), or in the muscle zone (indicating callosities), then one must not neglect to make a thorough examination of the mouth-throat area. Dark points in this area will suggest that the heart damage is secondary to a focal infection arising in the teeth or tonsils (angina, diphtheria).

7. *Coronary sclerosis:* was earlier the privilege of elderly and aged persons. Today, however, it not infrequently affects persons between 30 and 50 years of age. In the iris it is recognised by the following signs: At 15′ the iris-wreath shows a thicker white margin, conjoined with the lower arc of a cardiac weakness sign, and extending with it to the muscle zone. (See iris illus. 5.).

Sometimes a fine white line can be observed running obliquely from this white margin to the spleen area. This line is a sign of threatened cardiac infarct. (See iris illus. 6.)

8. *Roemheld syndrome:* is shown in the iris as a strong dilatation of the colon (i.e. iris-wreath) in the direction of the heart area. This dilatation may lie above or below the heart area. (See iris illus. 5, 6, 9, 12.)

9. *Coloured flecks in the heart area:* Such colour or toxin flecks in the heart area are small light to brownish-red pigment flecks. These indicate that the patient suffers mentally, and such patients tend strongly to brooding (melancholy, true depression, religious delusions, etc.). These signs very often go together with abdominal disturbances —usually affecting persons of Sepia-type (yellow glistening of the nose, dirty ring around the mouth, unable to get going in the mornings yet gay and lively in the evenings.)

The Blood Circulation

The arteries and veins refer changes affecting the whole system to the third lesser zone = Blood zone. In the observation of this zone special attention is given to light or dark colouring. A strong lightening of this zone over the entire iris indicates that the blood is heavily laden with uric acid; whereas a darkening, or several large usually somewhat obliterated weakness-signs, extending to the muscle zone, indicate general circulatory and muscle weakness. The patient feels tired, sleepy and inefficient (hypotonia).

Small dark point-like signs in the blood zone constitute a danger signal. They indicate that the state of the blood is not good. The protective function is lacking in that the leucocytes are no longer being adequately provided. In such a case, the patient should be warned before every proposed operation. Iris illustration 10 shows these dark spots distributed over the whole iris, as well as in the blood and muscle zones. The lymph glands are no longer able to function.

If the blood zone in the upper half of the iris is much lighter, while the lower half is dark, it indicates congestion of the head and ischaemia of the intestines. Reverse these signs in the iris, and there is ischaemia of the brain and hyperaemia of the abdomen.

In this chapter the condition of arteriosclerosis should be discussed, since in our civilised countries hardly anyone will escape its influence. It appears in all individuals sooner or later—more or less pronounced, and shows itself by affecting those organs which the mode of life has most strongly stressed. In the iris it is shown by whitish-grey to whitish-yellow deposits, mainly in the skin zone. Often this becomes an arcus senilis, a characteristic arc around the entire iris obscuring the iris structure. The arcus senilis enables one to assess the biological age of the patient concerned.

In the alcoholic, the arteriosclerosis ring is particularly strongly indicated in the areas for liver and spleen. With mental workers, it is marked in the brain sector. Where there is C-N-S sclerosis we find a sharp white neurasthenic ring clearly indicated. Coronary sclerosis has been described above under heart signs. (See iris illus. 5.)

Chapter 12

Diseases of the Respiratory Organs

(a) Nose—Left iris 52′, right iris 8′ approx.

(b) Throat and larynx—Left iris 45′–47′, right iris 13′–15′.

(c) Trachea—Right iris 12′–14′ only.

(d) Bronchi—Left iris 15′–17′, right iris 43′–45′.

(e) Lungs—Left iris 10′–15′, right iris 45′–50′ respectively, from the muscle zone outwards.

(f) Pleurae—Left iris and right iris, 15′–19′, 41′–45′. (Strictly speaking, the pleurae do not belong to the respiratory organs, but as is well known, are often disturbed together with the lungs, thus requiring them to be mentioned here.)

1. *Inflammation of the upper respiratory passages* ((a) to (c)): as may occur especially in the form of mucous membrane catarrh following chill—shows as white flakes or clouds in the specified areas. White wisps, running outwards to the iris margin, indicate an acute catarrhal discharge.

2. *Chronic catarrh of the upper respiratory organs:* is shown by dark grey wisp-signs.

3. *Lacunae* = weakness-signs: in the area for the upper respiratory passages, indicate a weakness of these organs and permanent catarrhal tendencies. More important than the signs in the areas for the upper respiratory passages are those which show in the area for bronchi, lungs and pleurae.

The bronchi very often became involved together with disturbances of the upper respiratory organ, in which case, the signs described above are also found in the bronchial areas.

Disturbances of the Lungs

One must not omit to look at the kidney areas, since lungs and kidneys have close connections with each other.

1. *Pneumonia* (inflammation of the lungs): in the muscle zone of the lung areas are seen distinct white clouds or wisps.

2. *Emphysema* (dilation of the lung): the lung area is dark and shows commencing lacunae (weakness-signs) extending outwards beyond the usual limits.

Every darkening in the lung areas is an expression of defective oxygen exchange, be it following acute emphysema, stasis from cardiac conditions, or merely reflective of poor breathing habits.

3. *Pertussis* (whooping cough): as with coughs from chill, whooping cough shows the usual white flakes or clouds in the appropriate areas during the early stages. In the convulsive stage it is evidenced by nerve rings which interrupt in the lung areas. After badly resolved whooping cough there remains a definite lung weakness, which shows as one or more large areas of darkening in the right iris at 40'–47'. These dark signs greatly resemble the lacunae (weakness-signs). If several of these signs are found in the lung and pleural areas (right 40'–47'), together with others occurring simultaneously in the lower nasal quadrant (right 15'–20'), then there is a hereditary disposition to asthma.

If these signs are also found in the left iris, together with cardiac weakness-signs, then the patient suffers from cardiac and pulmonary asthma. (See iris illus. 4, 5.)

4. *Pulmonary tuberculosis:* tuberculosis of the lung is hardly to be recognised on the basis of the lung signs alone. It is necessary here to search for other signs, especially in the intestinal zone, kidney area, and in the mucous membrane zone of the lung fields. In the intestinal zone, lying close to the iris-wreath, the so-called 'Schnabel-lacunae' may be found—these can also lie outside the iris-wreath. Important signs confirming the suspected lung T.B. are stasis signs in the left kidney area. (With dark kidney area, also look for the 'kidney-nail' = high arched finger nail.)

Further signs which give support to the diagnosis of lung T.B. are yellowish-white deposits in the mucous membrane zone of the lung areas. These can also appear in the form of small white clouds. A further sign is a very dark to black skin zone in this area. The deposit or clouds do not lie distributed in the manner typical of acute chill signs in the mucous membrane zone (arranged in arc form), but lie vertically one under the other in a straight line. In definite cases of lung T.B. the iris fibres in the lung area have the appearance of 'combed hair' (Maubach, Angerer). (See iris illus. 3, 7.)

Cavities are very difficult to recognise—as dark signs which are round at the bottom and flattened at the top, like a vertical section through a cup. In the dark grey sign lies a blacker point.

5. *Pulmonary carcinoma:* the signs for these conditions are very difficult to diagnose—especially for beginners. The signs are dark signs which extend in the width, and are not like the weakness-signs which are oval in length, since these signs become more oval in breadth. The dark sign seems to project forward from the depths of the iris. There is always a toxin-fleck nearby.

6. *Dry pleurisy:* shows fine white lines in the pleural area which extend outwards to the skin zone.

7. *Pleurisy with effusion:* is suggested by an inward deviation of the skin zone as a dark arc formation at left iris 15′–17′ or right iris 43′–45′. (See iris illus. 8.)

If simultaneously one finds light inflammation lines and small black signs in the back areas—left iris 43′, right iris 17′—then the danger of suppuration is indicated.

If the inflammation signs are prominent in profile, then a protracted condition is indicated, especially when the signs are to be seen in the left iris at 40′–45′ nasal segment. When with conditions of this kind the signs are apparent in profile, then the possibility of T.B. must always be considered.

8. *Pleural suppuration:* usually appears after acute pleurisy, but can also arise without evident cause. It shows as fine cobweb signs (transversales). (See iris illus. 8, 10.)

Chapter 13

Diseases of Kidney and Bladder

1. The Kidneys

The kidneys show their signs at right iris 28′–30′ and left iris 30′–32′, commencing directly against the iris-wreath and extending outwards to the fourth and fifth minor zones. The kidney is all the more healthy the less its area is indicated (Schulte).

If both kidneys register, then in many cases it is a question of overstrain, suggesting that the system is overladen with poisonous substances and that one or several other organs (intestines, skin and lungs) show conditions of functional insufficiency. In such cases one also finds an early or closed weakness-sign, or darkening of the kidney area.

True kidney disease usually takes place in one kidney only, and the following signs may be seen:

1. *Nephritis:* inflammation of the kidney. In acute conditions, small white points, wisps or clouds, or also small white streaks are found in the kidney area, which take on a yellowish colouring as the conditions become chronic. With older damage, the iris-wreath in the kidney area is contracted inwards. (See iris illus. 1, 2, 3, 4, 7 and 8.)

If the condition is one of cysto-pyelitis then sharp white lines or wisp signs are also found in the bladder area.

2. *Renal hypo-function:* functional weakness of the kidney. The kidney area shows a dark weakness-sign, which is markedly widened in the muscle zone. Patients with these signs pass scanty urine and have high-domed finger nails.

3. *Contracted kidney:* one finds in the kidney area dark to black points or streaks as signs of tissue disintegration. The condition is one of irreparable damage leading to progressive disturbance and renal insufficiency, with consequent uraemia. When these sharp black signs are seen, they are a reminder to be cautious (not dark wisps—these are signs of unresolved catarrh), and in addition to the customary urine analysis, to measure the blood pressure frequently, and also if possible

to observe the fundus of the eye. Other signs of contracted kidney are a weakness-sign in the heart area, and in addition to the small black kidney signs a large suprarenal sign.

4. *Renal stone*, nephrolithiasis: occurs more frequently than is generally accepted—it is not for certain established diagnostically in every case. For so long as concretions are retained in the renal pelvis no signs for stone can be found in the iris unless its presence results in inflammation of the mucous membrane—and this possibility is always there. When stimulation of the mucous membrane of the renal pelvis arises from concretions, one finds in the kidney area a small white streak (as distinct from the sign of inflammation arising otherwise: white clouds) close to the iris-wreath. These small white streaks disappear, however, when the inflammation recedes, and leave behind no sign of special significance. Such cases are only seldom seen by the irisdiagnostician, usually accidentally, when a patient comes on account of some other complaint. Generally, the condition is one of ureteral colic, without inflammation signs in the kidney or ureteral areas. Only a loosening of the iris fibres is to be seen in the organ area of the ureter: right iris 30′–35′, left iris 25′–30′.

When a sharp-edged stone lodges in the renal pelvis a local circumscribed inflammation first arises. This leads to the above-mentioned small white signs in the iris. If the condition in the renal pelvis results in damage to the mucous membrane and degeneration of tissue, then a small dark to black point-like sign develops in the white sign. These small injuries and inflammations heal quickly when the stone shifts to another position in the renal pelvis, so that from these repeated local injuries several small black points develop in the area for renal pelvis.

It would be untrue to infer that all such signs as have been discussed refer to renal gravel. My view is that a single stone can also give rise to such signs. Much depends upon the kind of stone, as to whether these signs will develop. These small point-like signs are not the only signs in the iris for stones. Sometimes we find several points surrounded by a thin white line, suggesting that frequent inflammatory response to stone damage of the renal pelvis has already occurred, and also that such has healed again.

One sometimes finds a black streak with a point on top. It looks like an upside down comma. Such a sign suggests that there is a large stone in the renal pelvis, which from its size and weight has resulted in an indentation of the renal tissues, destroying mucous membrane and connection tissues.

The signs described so far can exist without the patient complaining of, or having complained of painful symptoms in the kidney region. Where there are painful conditions one always finds a white sign (inflammation sign) by the black sign. According to the degree of inflammation, small white streaks or larger white clouds show, which may extend to the neighbourhood of the kidney areas. With extension of the inflammatory process, and destruction of the renal tissues, there will appear against the large white clouds several large, longish or zig-zag black signs. ((Black signs = tissue destruction = loss of substance.)

5. *Hydronephrosis,* renal stasis: arises as the result of pressure from inside or outside (stones, tumours, etc.), whereby the ureter is con-stricted and the urine collects in the renal pelvis, resulting in a consider-able dilatation of the renal pelvis. In the iris the condition is recognised by a wide separation of the iris fibres in the kidney area, with many long black signs which appear between the fibres. In well marked cases, the iris fibres are observed to be running in large arcs which extend over the extremity area (30′) and extend through the region for inguinal, uterine and rectal areas: right iris 25′, left iris 35′. (See iris illus. 7.)

6. *Floating kidney:* is recognised by a displacement of the kidney areas in the direction of the abdominal area. One sees a distinct white arc which extends out from the iris-wreath into the lower temporal quadrant of the iris. In addition, one often finds a contraction of the wreath at right iris 45′, or left iris 15–20′, which arises through pressure of the displaced kidney upon the intestine. (See iris illus. 2.)

Floating kidney and hydronephrosis have quite similar signs. They are easily distinguished by the long black signs (loss of substance) which are found with hydronephrosis but not with floating kidney.

7. It is important to draw attention to the close connection between lungs and kidneys (see also Chapter 12, Respiratory Organs). Thus, for example, there is no lung T.B. without kidney signs in the left iris. (Right iris: hereditary, left iris: acquired.)

2. The Bladder

A bladder sign is typically found in the fourth minor zone—the muscle zone, in the right iris at 22′, and in the left iris at 37′.

Bladder signs in the right iris are of organic origin and usually hereditary. Those in the left iris arise from infection. With bladder signs in the right iris one should give attention to signs in the ear areas, follow-ing the rule: Forefathers with bladder troubles—children with ear troubles. Children having dark bladder signs in the right iris are usually found to have signs in the ear area. Such children tend towards aural disturbances.

In the case of bladder signs in the left iris, look for an aortic sign. If both areas—bladder and aorta—are indicated, then consider the possibility of luetic infection. In such a case a heart sign is usually found as well.

1. *Cystitis:* inflammation of the bladder: shows white wisps, clouds or lines in the bladder area, or also a dark sign with a surrounding white border. If cramp occurs with bladder troubles (vesical spasm), then the appropriate area will show interrupted cramp-rings (contraction rings = nerve rings).

2. *Atony of the bladder:* is a muscular weakness and shows as dark oval lacunae or dark wisp signs in the fourth minor zone (muscle zone) of the bladder area.

3. *Cystic paralysis*—danger of: is indicated by an extension of this weakness-sign (lacuna) out over the fifth minor zone.

Chapter 14

Endocrine disorders and the Lymphatic system

1. Glands with Internal Secretions

Apart from the genital glands and the pancreas which have been described elsewhere, the following glands belong to the endocrine system:

   i. Pituitary
   ii. Pineal
   iii. Thyroid
   iv. Parathyroid
   v. Thymus
   vi. Suprarenal

i. *Pituitary:* which lies in the sella turcica, is recognisable by iris changes in the brain sector, locally as follows—right iris 60-2', left iris 58–60'—in the muscle zone.

There are no muscles in the brain, so the skeletal zone representing the base of the skull reaches as far as the blood zone. Thus, for example, in a case of fracture of the base of the skull the signs of damage are observed in the blood zone, here lying closer in towards the iris-wreath than would be the case with skeletal injuries of other parts. The bones of the cranial vault are represented in the skin zone.

The recognition of a disturbance of the pituitary is of greatest importance, since the pituitary is the regulator of all the remaining organs of internal secretion.

The disease-signs are shown as follows:

Lightening—as sign of over-activity, very often with a similar lightening in the areas for the corresponding sexual organs.

Darkening—as an expression of hypofunction, particularly affects the secondary sexual organs, giving rise to the clinical picture of hypophyseal obesity.

Pituitary tumours show clearly as dark tumour-signs extending widthwise, as is characteristic of tumours of other organs.

In the iris, the pituitary area lies opposite the suprarenal area, indicating the close connection between these two organs. When one of these glands is shown in the iris, indicating abnormal disturbance, then one considers the possibilities of cure. If both organs are registered (as in iris illus. 9) then the slightest condition must be attended to.

ii. *Epiphysis* (pineal): according to many other authors, the gland has its place in the iris according to the indication made on the topographical chart shown in Figure 10. I can give no iris sign for disturbance of this gland.

iii. *Thyroid gland:* shows in the right iris at approx. 14′–17′ and left iris 43′–46′ in the sixth minor zone. In the case of hyperfunction, a lightening of the area appears. A thyroid hypofunction is recognised by a darkening of the area.

Clinically, there is more or less a definite picture of myxoedema with hypofunction, which in its lighter forms is more widely distributed than is generally diagnosed. In thyroid disturbance the heart can register in sympathy, and the heart area must be thoroughly scrutinised. In most cases one finds lacunae, eventually in association with white lines. Therefore, appropriate cardiac medicinal support should not be omitted. A close connection also exists between the thyroid and the abdomen (Premenstrual syndrome).

iv. *Parathyroid glands:* as is well known, the parathyroid glands lie behind, or near to the thyroid glands, and so we also find the iris signs in the thyroid gland areas, rather nearer to the iris-wreath. The signs are very difficult to recognise. With these organs one rather relies upon the clinical symptoms of tetany: von Recklinghausens disease, and also the significance of the contraction-rings in the iris.

v. *Thymus gland:* the thymus gland shows its sign in the following areas—right iris 43′ approx., left iris 17′ approx.—in the fourth and fifth minor zones. In the same place, though rather more peripherally (fifth minor zone) lies the mammary gland position. One may easily distinguish these two signs since the mammary gland itself only develops fully when the thymus has atrophied.

vi. *Suprarenal glands:* these glands, whose functions have only in recent times been fully investigated, have their areas next to the kidney areas directly adjacent to the iris-wreath—right iris 30′–32′ approx., left iris 28′–30′ approx. If the suprarenal areas are lighter, then the indication is one of over-activity. We find these signs in rheumatic conditions together with an overlay in the entire muscle zone of whitish to yellowish clouds.

A dark weakness-sign (lacuna) in the suprarenal area indicates a suprarenal insufficiency. If these conditions have already occurred, one also finds besides the suprarenal sign, a lacuna in the heart area and a large dilatation of the iris-wreath. (See iris illus. 9—Left iris: Vegetative dystony.)

2. The Lymphatic System

Disease conditions of the lymphatic system show themselves almost everywhere in the iris. The signs are found in the iris-wreath, and in the fifth and sixth minor zones.

With encumbrance of the lymphatic apparatus the sixth zone appears strongly white to yellowish-white, as a general sign of over-activity. The most severe degree are found in the irides of persons of lymphatic constitution.

An overburdened lymphatic system is also shown by a thick white iris-wreath, with strongly marked white lines radiating to the mucous membrance zone, where they terminate as thick white clouds. These signs of hyperactivity are especially to be observed in infants and small children (nutritional errors). If the signs of hyperactivity become chronic we have such signs as are shown in iris illus. 1, 4, 6 and 8, e.g. mucous membrane catarrh, bronchial asthma, exudative diathesis, urticaria.

If a failure of the lymph system develops (leucopenia), then we see dark points in the iris lying dispersed throughout the whole of the ciliary zone. These points are not black, since there is no loss of substance. The sign indicates that the body's own defence mechanism is lacking. This condition is shown in iris illus. 10.

If dark points are seen in the blood zone, then this is a warning sign.

Particular attention is required in the case of female patients with regard to the mammary glands, whose signs lie in both irides. With women over 30 years of age the mammary areas should be carefully investigated for any developing tumour-sign.

Chapter 15

Diseases of the Spleen

The spleen has its area in the left iris, 20'–25' in the sixth minor zone. A lighter colour in the spleen area is found with inflammation of the spleen (splenitis), and also in diseases of stomach and intestine. A darkened spleen area indicates a diminished function of this organ. This is found with blood stasis following myocardial weakness, and with liver complaints.

The spleen and liver have a close connection to one another. Patients in whom spleen and liver areas are darkened cannot sleep at night. A very dark spleen area enables one to diagnose the tendency to feverish illnesses.

An enlarged spleen is suggested when the spleen area in the iris is enlarged, when the iris-wreath is contracted in towards the intestinal zone, or any existing cramp-rings are displaced inwards towards the iris-wreath.

At first, the tumour-signs in the spleen area are lighter, from the over-activity, but with functional insufficiency of the spleen, the spleen area becomes darkened and black points develop.

Chapter 16

Diseases of the Genital Organs

In disturbances of the male sexual organs the following iris signs are found:

i. Urethra: right iris 23', left iris 37' approx.—outwards from the bladder area.

ii. Prostate gland: in both irides between the areas for bladder and urethra, thus—right iris 23' and left iris 37'—in the second and third major zones.

iii. Testicles and epididymis: right iris 35' and left iris 25'— in the third major zone.

iv. Seminal vesicles: right iris 25'.

(a) Inflammatory and Irritable Conditions

According to Schulte, a fine white streak in the area for urethra in the right iris is the sign for acute venereal disease. With chronicity of the disease the sign becomes yellow to grey, and then also shows in the left iris. White wisps or clouds from the bladder area to the iris rim, when they appear in both irides, indicate an inflammation of the prostate. If the white signs are already present in the bladder area, then the condition is one of cystic and urethral catarrh.

In sexual over-stimulation, white wisps are found in all sex organ areas, including that for testicle.

Sexual overstimulation or masturbation can be assumed, when in the left eye a blood-vessel runs over the sclera to the area for rectum and to the area for testicle (ovary).

(b) Insufficiency and Sclerosis

Dark signs—grey to dark wisps, clouds or lines—also testify to an under-function or weakness of the affected sexual organs. Small black points, or grey-black indented marks, are signs for sclerosis, i.e. enlargement. These signs are especially found in the area for prostate gland.

Iris signs in conditions of the female sexual organs: One finds:

    i. Ovary: right iris 35′ and left iris 25′—in the third major zone.

    ii. Uterus: right iris 25′—in the second major zone.

    iii. Vagina: right iris 25′–28′—in the third major zone.

The ovaries, as with the testicles in man, have close connections with the fore-brain. In case of inflammation-signs in the area for ovary (white signs), one often finds similar signs in the opposite brain area. The same may occur with the dark signs of under-activity, where we often find the so-called Brain-Ovary line. The appearance of this line always indicates disturbance of the sex life with effects upon the cerebrum and mind. Patients with such signs are depressed and oppressed.

In this connection, one should refer to the hypotrophic state and deficient development of the internal and external sex organs in both sexes. This condition may be presumed when one finds a patient with short flat finger-nails. In such cases, the deficient development of the ovary affects the nerve life of the fore-brain, giving rise to the following symptoms—

Frontal headache, giddiness, disturbance from exposure to the sun, travel sickness, sense of pressure from headwear, bitten finger-nails and enuresis in children.

All these symptoms can be confirmed, either singly or in association, in persons with flat short finger-nails. Short nails frequently recede behind the fingertips, especially when they are continuously bitten off or torn off. This is pathological, and no child should be punished for the condition. Headaches cease after the menopause. Furthermore, it is found with especially small nails that there are small dimunitive nipples with deficient lactation in childbirth. On the other hand, nature makes up for these deficiencies by giving an easy normal digestion, so that these persons are seldom thin. Usually, they are of a simple homely disposition, a probable consequence of the influenced cerebral function.

Ovarian tumours (mostly cysts) are shown by broad dark signs = tumour signs. In such cases one must also note the iris-wreath, which is compressed inwards towards the pupil in that area.

If the ovarian sectors are shown wide and dark, then it is probable that the menopause will occur prematurely. It is of interest here to note that women whose left ovary was removed usually cannot have any more children.

A white discharge-sign in the area for uterus, which generally extends to the iris rim, is the sign for an acute uterine catarrh and resultant discharge.

A dark discharge-sign indicates a condition of chronic uterine catarrh. (See iris illus. 3.)

If one finds a dark line drawn through the middle of the uterus area, then the patient is likely to suffer from 'flushes', which usually first appear in the pre-climacterium and the climacterium. The sign may also be found in younger women, and this will confirm any question of the appearance of such 'flushes'.

Displacement of the uterus is recognised by the fact that the iris fibres in the uterus-area run in large strongly curved arcs enclosing dark lines. The iris fibres then reach as far as the kidney area. With a uterus displaced towards the rectum (retroversion) there is a displacement of the iris fibres from 22' to 20'—therefore to the low back area, and since there is often pressure upon the rectum, the above signs may also be seen in the left iris in the rectum area. Where there is prolapse the dark uterus sign extends lower and often reaches as far as the iris-rim. (See iris illus. 11.)

Uterine neoplasms are recognisable in the early stages often only by changes in the iris wreath. Therefore it is absolutely essential to observe any deviation of the wreath upwards, since with all new formations in the abdominal cavity, especially of the larger kind, such as ovarian cysts and uterine fibroids, an indentation of the iris-wreath develops, even when no true sign of swelling has yet appeared. In the subsequent development of the disease, the typical widthwise dark tumour-sign forms in the affected organ area.

In contrast to the large tumours, the uterine carcinoma shows at first only in the form of very small, somewhat pin-head size dark points, around which the iris fibres separate. Only if the condition deteriorates, and disturbs the normal body tissues do these points become black.

Small black points with small white transverse lines in the area for uterus are generally the consequence of difficult childbirth (lesions of the cervix).

If cramp-rings are found which interrupt in the uterus area, the patient complains of painful cramps during the menstrual period.

In the iris, the cerebellum lies opposite the uterus (cerebellum-uterus line), and both these organs have a close relation to one another. Patients in whom the cerebellum-uterus line is indicated tend towards hysteria—they are noisy and talk too much. On the other hand, patients showing the cerebellum-rectum line (left iris) tend to hypochondria.

Patients with such signs are silent, say almost nothing, and bear their sorrows without much complaint.

The appearance of the uterus sign in the left iris is very much disputed. On this point I cite Phil. Jung: 'Since both vagina and penis as single organs are found in both irides, why should the uterus be an exception?' Jung found that with severe genital conditions the uterus signs appear in both irides, whereas in slighter conditions only the right iris shows the sign, and, as he says, this may have its origin in the strong 'positivity' of the uterus as a developed organ.

Chapter 17

Disorders of the Spinal Column

The spinal area lies in the right iris 15'–22' and in the left iris 37'–45'—in the fifth minor zone. White signs in these areas indicate inflammation and pain. In the case of spinal changes, such as damaged intervertebral disc, one sees white lines which run outwards from the iris-wreath. If the damage has existed for some time, dark lines in addition to the white lines are seen or dark to black points in the skeletal zone, especially in the areas for cervical and lumbar spine. These two regions of the spine lie diametrically opposite to one another in the iris. (Note: Axilla-Loin line.) The pupil in this area is often flattened and/or the iris-wreath is displaced towards the pupil. (See iris illus. 12.)

Multiple sclerosis is a disturbance of the brain and spinal cord, where the pathology leads to vascular changes and to a degeneration of nerve tissue, in which case connective tissue (hyperplasia of neuroglia) appears. Corresponding to the different regions of the brain and spinal cord affected in this disease, iris signs can appear in the spinal area, cervical area, as well as in the area for medulla oblongata. In such conditions one finds several black small points which lie one under the other.

In contrast to the intervertebral disc injuries, in which usually only one black point is found, and where also small meandering veins run in over the sclera to the corresponding spinal areas, the condition of multiple sclerosis always shows several small points, and the blood vessel picture on the sclera is missing. Next to the signs in the spinal areas or medulla, in cases of multiple sclerosis signs of over-activity affecting the sexual organs and rectum are also found.

Chapter 18

Disease Signs in the Cranial Areas

The head takes in the whole of the upper half of the iris except for the inclusion of heart and lungs. The important organs here include the mouth with the teeth and tonsils, nose and forehead with their accessory sinuses, the eye, brain and ear.

The areas for teeth and accessory sinuses deserve special attention since they are frequently the seat of disseminating or latent foci, which are seen as small black points. With latent foci, one sees on the sclera small tortuous venules which run to the affected area and have at their ends small bluish shining nodes. With disseminating foci the vessels go up to the iris, and with acute inflammations even on to the iris.

The areas for eyes—right iris 7′, left iris 53′—and the areas for ears, right iris about 52′, left iris 8′—are lighter in colour if there have been previous inflammatory conditions. White wisps or clouds are seen, which for example, in the case of purulent inflammation of the middle ears, extend to the outermost iris rim. These acute states are so easily established clinically that one seldom needs to make an exact iris-diagnosis for otitis media. With such disturbances also pay attention to the vascular state of the sclera. Much more frequently, however, one finds in these areas dark signs in the form of dark streaks, and this suggests an old injury which has not completely healed. If, however, these black streaks go inwards towards the iris-wreath, then there may be an optic nerve or auditory nerve weakness, and the patient complains of visual or auditory disturbances.

The brain area in both irides extends from 58′-7′, encompassing a large space, and assuming a correspondingly great importance. A much lighter colour of the brain areas suggests a congestion of blood in the brain, often accompanied by vertigo. White, or in the case of a brown stomach zone—brownish, radiating lines which run from the stomach zone to the brain area are signs for headache, whose origin lies in an over-activity of the stomach.

Single fine white lines in the brain area, the so-called nerve lines, indicate an over-activity of the head and brain nerves with neuralgic pains. Small ring-formations of whitish points in the fifth minor zone (resembling a string of small wax pearls) are signs for circulatory disturbance of the head, which the patient experiences as a feeling of numbness.

Darkening of the brain area in any case suggests a circulatory disturbance, which in such a case is attended by tiredness, depression, weakness and dizziness consequent upon the defective brain circulation —usually the result of cardiac weakness.

If lacunae are to be seen in the brain area then one may assume weakness of thought power and intelligence.

Dark signs in the area for cerebellum in the right iris indicate an hereditary disposition to epilepsy (according to Frau Madaus). If the signs appear in the left iris, it is supposed to indicate weakness of will through faulty upbringing. If radii solaris, dark radiating furrows, are seen in the iris running from the pupil to the brain area, then there is a state of cerebral weakness. In the remainder of the iris they signify nerve weakness of the organs to which they run, more especially exhaustion of the C-N-S. When they radiate out from the iris-wreath only, exhaustion of the vegetative nervous system is indicated.

Chapter 19

The Autonomic Nervous System in the Iris

The question arises: Is it true that the sympathetic nervous system registers in the iris as a square, as shown in several iris charts?

After studying the existing systems, I have come to the conclusion that the sympathetic trunk and the sympathetic ganglia have their proper place around the iris-wreath, but before giving my interpretation, I would like to outline the relevant observations given in these systems.

Schlegel writes as follows in his book *Die Augendiagnose des Dr. Ignatz von Peczely*, 4th edition, published by Verlag Krüger and Co., Leipzig, 1924:

> Irisdiagnosis has been greatly enriched by Anderschou's location of the ganglionic plexi in the iris. He portrays the ganglionic plexus as a chainlike range of elevations between the nutritive organ areas (stomach and intestines) and the other organ areas of the body. Observation of it in the iris is rather difficult, and not possible in an iris of compact and dense texture.
>
> On close examination with a lens, the small indications are found in conjunction with the organ-arcs. A part of the colon and intestines is to be found inside the sympathetic line, but all borders are dependent upon the mutual influences of the affected (diseased) parts. In this connection, I should like to point out that the medulla oblongata also has its place here.

In the Anderschou chart, the sympathetic line is indicated as a square around the iris-wreath, with arcs of different sizes directed inwardly and outwardly.

In his book *Der Krankheitsbefund aus den Augen*, 3rd revised edition 1920, Peter Johannes Thiel writes thus on the solar plexus:

The solar plexus, a ganglionic plexus of the general nervous system, is also the control centre of the body-life, which through the umbilical cord has built up the whole body according to the three polar axes of the three dimensions. The animal nervous system, subject to consciousness and will, has its centre in the brain. The control centre of the vegetative nervous system corresponds in the iris with the central fibrous ring of the pupillary sphincter around the pupil.

So much for Peter Johannes Thiel. On plates 1 and 2 of his book the solar plexus is indicated around the pupil in the stomach zone. Individual nerve plexi, such as the heart, kidney and liver plexus, he places around the square-shaped intestinal section.

Kronenberger, in his book *Die Irisdiagnostik*, 5th edition, published by Verlag W. Schmitz, Giessen, June 1949, writes:

The position of the solar plexus (plexus coeliacus) has been defined by only two or three investigators, who, however, are very vague in their exact location, and with whom I must completely disagree. According to the anatomical position, the solar plexus is found in front of the sympathetic trunk, in which case it is unquestionably a gastro-intestinal plexus. In spite of other opinion, it can only be placed with the sympathetic nervous system, whose location in the iris-wreath surrounding the digestive area, therefore the intestinal area, is quite definite. The sympathetic trunk shows as a ring-formation around the solar plexus in the region of the iris-wreath.

He correlates the Vagus with the upper layer of the iris, the Sympathetic with the second layer, and the motor and sensory nerve fibres with the third layer. The correspondence with Hense's view of the nerve layers is significant.

Kronenberger's interpretation of the threefold arc-formation and the nerve rings is found in Hense in a different form. This interpretation of the three arc-formations has presumably also led to the introduction of the three major, six minor regions in the iris chart of Madaus-Flink. This division is easily seen in illustration 35 in the *Textbook of Organdiagnosis* by Kronenberger. However, he does not show a square-shaped iris-wreath.

Frau Magdelene Madaus has also indicated the sympathetic nervous system as a square in her *Lehrbuch der Irisdiagnose*, 3rd revised edition of 1926. She writes, however, that the sympathetic nervous system is not seen as a square, but that if signs such as black streaks or white lines go from the outer edge of the iris to the iris-wreath, or radiate out from the pupil and break through the iris-wreath, such signs always refer to the Sympathetic. It indicates that the complaints have a chronic character and would be difficult to cure.

In his book *Die Augendiagnose*, published 1927, Baumhauer describes the anatomical position of the sympathetic nervous system and its ramifications throughout the body. He reproduces the illustration as taken over from Anderschou by Schlegel, showing a square with the individual nerve plexi marked in.

H. Hence, in his *Heilsystem Truw*, 1931 edition, on Information Chart II, shows the Vagus and Sympathetic, the principal nerve centres and ganglia, in the iris-wreath, from which all organs are supplied.

Karl Huter, in his book *Illustriertes Handbuch der praktischen Menschenkenntnis*, Karl Huter Verlag, Althofnass bei Breslau, 1910, shows an iris chart in which the sympathetic nervous system is indicated around the iris-wreath as a square, and on which he marks the lower line as the sympathetic ganglia, and the upper line as the sympathetic nervous system with connections to the head. Although the organ areas do not quite correspond with the modern chart, one must agree that even at that time a good understanding had been worked out. Everything is so arranged that it could be developed further, thus enabling later investigators to improve the existing system.

There remains to be mentioned Dr. Bernard Jensen, U.S.A., who in his book, also places the vegetative nervous system around the iris-wreath.

In the works of the more recent investigators, Maubach, Angerer and Deck, we find no localisation of the vegetative nervous system.

After concluding this review of different authors and of the anatomical relations, I think I can claim that the following key to the location of the vegetative nervous system in the iris is in accordance with the findings of many investigators.

The autonomic nervous system is described as a nervous system which functions according to its own laws. Anatomically considered, the autonomic nervous system, together with the glands of internal secretion and the body fluids, forms a functional unity.

The Vagus (= Parasympathetic) is the 10th cranial nerve. It is also called the pneumogastric nerve. It consists of all those vegetative nerve fibres, including their origins and central connections, which arise in the mid-brain and the medulla oblongata, as well as in the sacral division. As the cranio-sacral system, it is functionally opposed to the thoracico-lumbar system (Sympathetic). The fibres of the parasympathetic do not run over the sympathetic trunk, but use true brain and spinal cord nerves as conductors.

The Sympathetic system, also known as the thoracico-lumbar system or the sympathetic trunk, has its cells of origin in the lateral horns of the thoracic and upper lumbar spinal cord. The spinal centres belonging to the vertebral column and spinal cord are subject to the influence of higher centres in the medulla oblongata, in the mid-brain, and in the cerebral cortex.

Solar Plexus—Coeliac plexus: the sympathetic fibres to the abdominal viscera do not arborise in the sympathetic trunk, but run within medullated sheaths to distant ganglia which lie in the posterior abdominal wall around the aorta and its branches, between pancreas, stomach and liver. These ganglia are connected with each other by numerous nerve fibres, the whole forming a radial structure which has been named Solar plexus. From this plexus, nerve fibres are supplied to the stomach, liver, pancreas, kidneys, adrenals, and upper intestinal viscera. The ganglia also receive nerve fibres from the sympathetic trunk.

The iris-wreath, as the border surrounding the stomach and intestinal zones, indicates that this should in some way represent the taking up of nutrient products from the digestive organs into the blood and lymph circulation. If we remember the anatomical position of the sympathetic trunk and the ganglia of the sympathetic nervous system, we must conclude that the iris-wreath is the only possible localisation for these nervous structures, with the fibres radiating towards the pupil to represent the function of the stomach and intestines, and the fibres radiating outwards to the ciliary margin representing all other body organs.

As to whether the sympathetic and vagus fibres can be differentiated into layers, as stated by Hense and Kronenberger, will have to remain undecided. It will be otherwise with the principal centres and ganglia and I believe that these can be localised more precisely in the iris. (See Figure 11.)

In the case of the Vagus, the supply to the wall of the trunk and to the extremities has its origin in an unknown centre in the spinal cord. For the viscera, there are two widely separated parasympathetic centres. The upper centre, which arises from three nuclei in the brain stem, innervates the head, thorax and intestines as far as the rectum. These three nuclei should be found in the iris in the 5th minor zone (Bone-zone): in the right iris at 50′–55′, and in the left iris at 5′–10′. The remaining centre, in the lowest section of the spinal cord (sacral outflow), is also to be found in the iris in the 5th minor zone (Bone-zone): in the right iris at 20′–25′, and in the left iris at 35′–40′.

Each terminal ganglion of the Vagus is located in the wall of the organ itself; not, as with the Sympathetic, in the sympathetic trunk. It must therefore be located in the appropriate organ area.

The Sympathetic nervous system, consisting of the sympathetic trunk and its ganglionic system, is divided into several principal supply areas. From the upper two ganglia, which lie in the neck and chest region, fibres are supplied to the head and to all thoracic organs. These are located in the iris on the iris-wreath at 42′–60′ and 1′–18′ in both irides.

The fourth principal ganglion (Coeliac ganglion = Solar plexus) influences the stomach and intestines, together with the fifth upper abdominal ganglion and the sixth lower abdominal ganglion. Therefore the stomach and intestinal areas (1st and 2nd minor zones) between the pupil and the iris-wreath are indicated. However, such organs as liver, pancreas, spleen, kidneys, and suprarenal bodies, are supplied from the solar plexus. We therefore find the indications in the iris at the iris-wreath, in the respective organ sectors. The bladder and the genitalia are innervated from the sixth lower abdominal ganglion, and the iris signs are similarly located in the respective organ areas.

If some particular section of the iris-wreath shows contraction or dilatation, then in my view, a disturbance of the corresponding ganglion and its efferent fibres is indicated. Further, one may presume that the organic disturbances are transmitted by the sympathetic fibres to the appropriate ganglion, ultimately resulting in damage, and hence—iris signs.

Although the square indication of the sympathetic nervous system seen in several iris-charts probably arose from purely schematic considerations, it may also have arisen partly from the fact that one finds a square-shaped iris-wreath in many irides. Such a sign implies the presence of a grave condition, and if occurring in both irides, indicates that a cure is no longer possible. The square iris-wreath suggests that a severe disturbance exists in the vegetative functions. Moreover, every practitioner will know that if an organ which has its location far away from the wreath gives rise to a sign which points towards the wreath, or even breaks through it, then damage to the vegetative nervous system must be considered.

Contraction or dilatation of the iris-wreath is associated with disturbance of the vegetative nervous system. If radiating white lines are present, it is necessary to decide whether they originate from the pupillary margin or from the iris-wreath. It can thus be recognised whether the complaints arise from disturbance of the vegetative nervous system (iris-wreath), or have a connection with the central nervous system (pupillary margin). Just as we consider whether the radii-solaris have their origin at the pupillary margin (= C.N.S.) or iris-wreath (= A.N.S.)

In my opinion, the terminal ramifications of the fibres of the two components of the autonomic nervous system (Vagus and Sympathetic), may only be distinguished by correlating the Vagus with the upper iris layer, and the Sympathetic with the second iris layer. In this respect, the observations of Hense and Kronenberger come nearest to the true facts.

According to the explanations of Dr. Walter Lang, Heidelberg, the correlation of the vegetative nervous system with the three layers of the iris cannot be proved. In his book *Die anatomischen und physiologischen Grundlagen der Augendiagnostik*, published by Karl F. Haug Verlag, Ulm/Donau, 1954, Lang has exhaustively described all possibilities of demonstration. He has weighed all the evidence, and assessed the arguments for and against. His work is the first serious attempt to give a scientific basis to Irisdiagnosis.

What conclusions are now to be drawn from the above considerations? Anatomically considered, the eye is a sphere, and the iris is a round disc with a central aperture. If the entire human body, consisting of a cylindrical trunk with several appendages, is to be projected into the round iris-disc, then it can only be portrayed as a circular topography with insertions for the appendages (extremities).

On this basis, it is not possible to accept that the intestinal area, or the nervous system, could in health be seen as a square, as shown in certain charts. If, however, a displacement of the normal iris structure is found, then it is to be considered as a sign for a disease condition. It is only possible to make a diagnosis from such changes in the structure and colour of the iris.

Chapter 20

Pigment Deposits in the Iris

The colour-signs in the iris, showing the deposition of pigments, are divided according to shape and colour. With regard to these conspicuous signs, there are three groups of pigments to be considered:

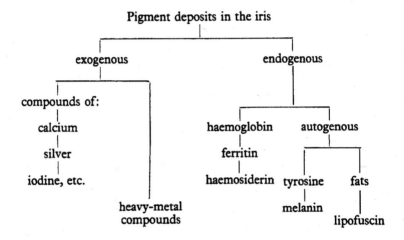

The endogenous pigments are important for iridology. To these endogenous pigments belong those of the haemoglobin group with the end-product haemosiderin (colour: red to brown), the melanin group (colour: brown to black), and lipofuscin, also referred to as the 'wear and tear' pigment (colour: light yellow to dark brown).

The melanin group of pigments have their origin in special dendron cells, melanocytes (also described as melanodendrocytes). These cells derive from the embryonic neural crest. The melanin originates in the melanocytes by means of complicated enzymatic processes. A first stage of melanin is the colourless amino-acid Tyrosine. This compound is transformed by the action of Tyrosinase through dihydroxyphenyl-alamine (DOPA) into melanin.

Melanin formation is also subject to hormone control. The pituitary gland secretes a melanocytotrophic hormone (MTH, also called melanocyte-stimulating hormone: MSH), which has a stimulating effect, while the adrenal hormones from the cortex and medulla appear to check the pigmentation process. From these different influences affecting the formation of pigment, it can be accepted that disturbances may give rise to a wide variation of manifestations within the total organism.

Melanin tends to migrate within the body. Because of its poor solubility as such, melanin is taken up by the cells of the reticulo-endothelial system, the melanophores, by a process of phagocytosis, and conveyed to wherever it supposedly serves some purpose. Melanin is found in the vicinity of inflammatory processes, and also with skin conditions accompanied by inflammation. Pigment migration also arises in the vicinity of tumors and within many tumorous conditions, e.g., melanosarcoma. One is also reminded of ulcerations of the lower leg, where melanin deposits occur over large areas.

It should also be mentioned here that melanin is found within the body as a normal constituent of the hair, skin and the posterior surface of the iris. It accumulates in the skin as a protection from the ultra-violet rays of the sun, where the melanin protects the skin from the carcinogenic effects of these rays.

If melanin deposits are found on the anterior surface of the iris, then there is a positive indication of the existence of serious metabolic disturbances. Indeed, according to the accompanying signs in the iris, one may speak of a pre-cancerous condition of the corresponding organs or systems which can ultimately lead to a cancerous state.

The iron-containing pigment: haemosiderin (haemofuscin) is a red-dish colour to begin with, and may then change towards dark brown (the colour change of a piece of rusting iron!). On the destruction of large quantities of red blood corpuscles, this pigment becomes deposited within the tissues of the body. It can also appear in the iris following internal or concealed haemorrhage. In my opinion it is not a sign for haemorrhagic tendencies, but only the sign of a large destruction of red blood corpuscles in which the iron is deposited in the tissues.

Lipofuscin: the 'wear and tear' pigment

This Fe-free pigment can appear in the iris in a range of colours varying from light yellow to black-brown. It is formed within the ganglion cells of the Nucleus niger and Locus ceruleus, and appears mostly as 'wear and tear' pigment in old age. However, it can also originate from protein metabolism without such regressive changes.

Lipofuscin (never melanin) is a constituent of the extra-pyramidal system. In the Zona reticularis of the suprarenal body, lipofuscin can be recognised microscopically as a dark brown colouring in conditions of old age. Although lipofuscin is described as a product of old age, it can also exist as a degeneration product in young people and as a sign of exhaustion of particular organs, hence the terms: liver-, renal- and pancreas-pigment.

At this point, I would like to include the group of rheumatic-gouty deposits. In my view, the duration of the condition can be assessed from the colour of the signs. The longer the disease has been present, the darker is the colour of the pigment.

Even though the above-mentioned pigments are topolabile, the presence of the flecks in the different zones of the iris can still be assigned to definite organ systems. If the light reddish pigment, as described in detail in the literature under the term—Nux vomica pigment, appears in the stomach and intestinal zone (first major zone), then it shows that a condition of fermentation affects these organs. If the discolouration extends outwards beyond the iris-wreath, then other organ systems can be affected.

The yellow to brown deposits which extend from the iris-wreath to the outer margin of the iris (Berberis pigment) indicate general disease of the body (Maubach: Reibekuchen-iris). In this case, the condition arises from a gouty disposition of hereditary origin. Indications of the acute phases of gout appear white, and generally lie next to dark signs in the bone area (fifth minor zone).

The pigments described as liver-, renal- and pancreas-pigment are likewise found in the ciliary zone.

Pigment deposits may appear in the iris if an organ is affected. However, since the differences of colour and localisation of pigment-flecks are insufficient for diagnosis, one must look for other signs in the organ areas of the iris in order to reach a definite opinion. Iridologists have been concerned with iris pigment-signs from the first beginnings of irisdiagnosis, commencing with Liljequist and continuing with Attila von Peczely, Schnabel and Angerer. In spite of their extensive works, there still remains a wide field for further research.

Chapter 21

Pupil Variations

The pupil as such is entirely dependent upon the function of the iris. Therefore, all reactions and conditions of the pupil are to be considered basically as no more than changes affecting the inner margin of the iris. For the irisdiagnostician, however, only those abnormal conditions are significant which by paralysis or irritation of the nerves controlling the muscles of the iris, produce changes in the function or state of the pupil. (M. sphincter pupillae = pupil contraction and M. dilatator pupillae = pupil dilation.) Consequently, all those disturbances which are caused by local injuries or other conditions of the eyeball are to be ignored.

The normal shape of the pupil is circular. It should lie in the centre of the iris (perhaps somewhat disposed towards the nasal side), and appear neither too large nor too small under ordinary conditions of lighting. The normal diameter is 3–4 mm. On the whole, relatively larger pupils are found in small children, while in adults the size of the pupil progressively diminishes as old age advances.

The pupil should not show any undue variation in width, and the movements of contraction and dilation should affect both pupils symmetrically.

Classification of Pupillary Phenomena

The pathological variations in the shape of the pupil may be divided into three groups:

1. Deformations:
   (a) Oval distortion,
   (b) Segmental flattening of the margin,
   (c) Local outward bulging,
   (d) Local inward bulging,
   (e) Degeneration of the edge of the pupil.

2. Variations in pupil diameter:
  (*a*) Miosis = symmetrical contraction of the pupils,
  (*b*) Mydriasis = symmetrical dilation of the pupils,
  (*c*) Anisocoria = inequality of pupils in size.
3. Discolouration of the pupil (so-called):
  (*a*) grey—caract,
  (*b*) green—glaucoma.

Total Deformations

Symmetrical deformations of the pupil are those in which the natural circular form deviates towards an oval shape. Such oval pupils may have similar or dissimilar axes of inclination, which may occur at all angles. These deviations are principally classified as vertical, horizontal, inclined parallel to left or right, and as upper or lower diverging ellipses.

Vertical ovals provide a sign of imminent sudden death (very shortly if the sign appears symmetrically in both irides, but at a longer interval if appearing in one eye only).

Oblique oval pupils are seen in patients who have tendencies towards psychic disturbance, more severe depression, and even to suicide (see Disharmony line).

If the vertical oval is to be considered as representing the effects of the head (brain) upon the lower half of the body, then the horizontal oval similarly illustrates the connection between the thyroid gland and the heart and lungs (angina pectoris with tendency to infarct, or asthma and respiratory paralysis, hormone influences).

In general, one can probably say that in the majority of cases, oval pupils indicate hereditary or acquired predisposition to apoplexy. However, in viewing the iris, one must ensure that an apparently oval shape of the pupil does not arise from an oblique view on the part of the observer.

Partial Deformations of the Pupils

On the whole, these deformations consist of localised flattenings and bulgings of the margin of the pupil. In this case one should note whether these distortions appear in the right or left eye, and whether they are found in the upper, lower, nasal or temporal sectors. A sunken condition of a flattened segment leads to inward bulging, corresponding to an increase of all symptoms.

All asymmetrical deformations of the pupil are reliable indications for assessing the condition of the nervous system, as well as to imply a disease condition of those organs whose areas are localised in the sector corresponding to the flattened segment. This second point is very important.

Flattening of the left pupil margin in the upper sector indicates psychic disturbances. Flattening of the lower sector of both pupils indicates severe muscle weakness affecting the legs.

Flattening of the pupil margin in the nasal sector indicates disturbance arising from the spinal cord and its nerve trunks, and includes physical and mental conditions. Temporal flattening corresponds more with hormone disturbances. From cerebellum to gonads, including suprarenals, pancreas and heart, these organs stand in close hormonal relationship. From this arises the clinical picture of vegetative dystony.

Flattening of the pupil margin in the upper sector of the right iris is more often seen in conditions associated with hysteria, whereas involvement of the same sector of the left iris indicates a predominance of melancholic states (see also right iris: Uterus-Cerebellum line, and left iris: Rectum-Cerebellum line).

Right temporal sector flattening suggests disturbance of the liver and consequent effects. In this case, the patients are suffering from liver encumbrance arising from hereditary preconditions caused by faulty nutrition and mode of life

Pathological Degrees of Pupil Size

An excessively contracted pupil is a sign for over-stimulation of the vegetative nervous system (vagotonia), whereas a widely dilated pupil indicates exhaustion of the vegetative nervous system (sympatheticotonia).

Anisocoria generally arises on a background of hereditary luetic damage, if there is no history of diphtheria or meningitis.

The so-called Discolourations of the Pupil

Since the pupil is merely a circular opening in the iris it cannot really be described as discoloured, but the underlying lens gives rise to the impression of colour change. Clinically, the grey discolourations (cataract) are to be distinguished from the green (glaucoma).

The grey discolouration can assume very different shapes, which according to Angerer and Schnabel may have variable causes. The principal causes are diabetes and arteriosclerosis. In the case of green discolouration, it is necessary to distinguish primary and secondary glaucoma.

Apart from these discolourations, signs of different shape may appear over the pupil. These may represent the remains of the foetal pupillary membrane, which originate from the iris-wreath as an irregular network of fine threads, and deposit as granules over the area of the pupil. These signs are supposed to suggest tuberculosis in the forebears.

Phenomena of the Edge of the Pupil (The 'neurasthenic' ring)

The margin of the pupil, pars iridica retinae, in its dilatation, colour, shape and plasticity, is a reflection of the central nervous system. One which is of delicate appearance, of reddish-brown colour and with a uniform edge, is to be regarded as normal. To enumerate the varieties of individual form and colour is beyond the scope of the present work.

Any signs in the corresponding sector of the iris should be interpreted in association with all phenomena affecting the margin of the pupil. As stated elsewhere, signs which displace or break through the iris-wreath refer to the vegetative nervous system. If such signs go out from the pupil or go through to reach the pupil, they refer to the central nervous system. Where signs relating to the organ areas extend to the pupillary margin, an edge-sign will be found. This sign differs in form and colour according to the nature of the disturbance.

One must always bear in mind that the eye represents a unity, and should be considered in its entirety. From this it follows that neither the edge of the pupil nor the peripheral margin of the iris alone can provide the basis for any diagnosis.

Figure 1

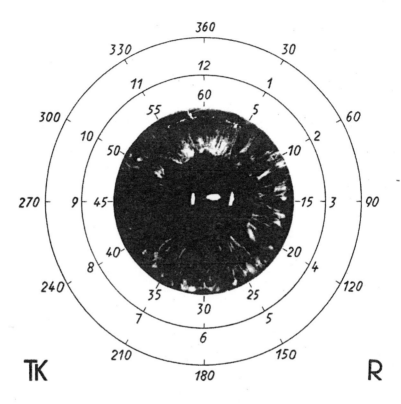

Schematic representation of the radial division of the iris into 360 degrees, 12 hours and 60 minutes.

Figure 2

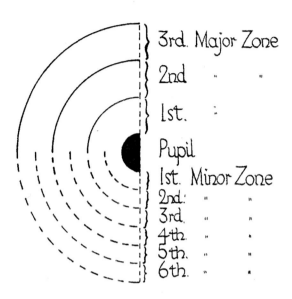

3rd. Major Zone

2nd　　　"　　　"

1st.　　:

Pupil

1st. Minor Zone

2nd.　"　　"

3rd.　"　　"

4th.　"　　"

5th.　"　　"

6th.　"　　"

Schematic representation of the circular division of the iris into three
major and six minor zones.

RIGHT IRIS

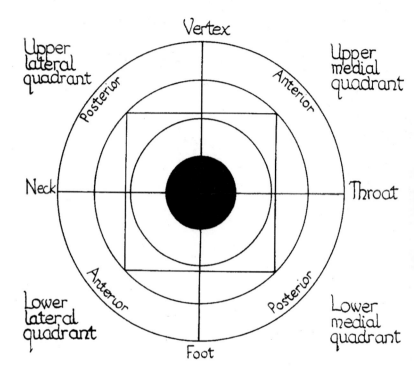

Schematic representation of the division of the iris into quadrants, and the Sympathetic-quadrant according to Schlegel.

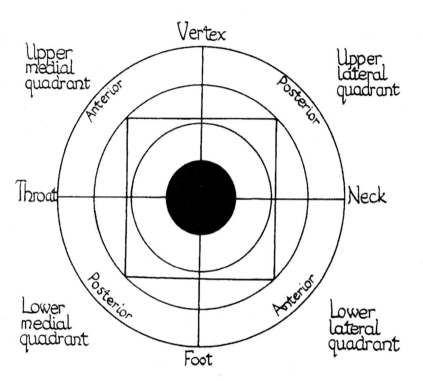

Figure 3

LEFT IRIS

Vertex

Upper medial quadrant

Anterior

Upper lateral quadrant

Posterior

Throat

Neck

Posterior

Lower medial quadrant

Anterior

Lower lateral quadrant

Foot

Frau Magdalene Madaus devotes a whole chapter to this Sympathetic-quadrant in her textbook on Irisdiagnosis.

RIGHT IRIS

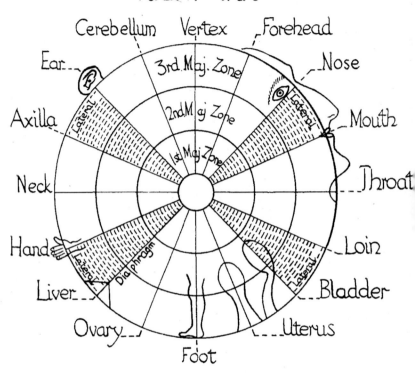

Schematic representation of the iris in 16 sectors:

Vertex line ⎫
Foot line ⎬ Equilibrium line.

Throat line ⎫
Neck line ⎬ Change-over line, also Disharmony line.

Nose line ⎫
Diaphragm line ⎬ Acute inflammation and pain line.

Ear line ⎫
Bladder line ⎬ Iufection line.

Figure 4

LEFT IRIS

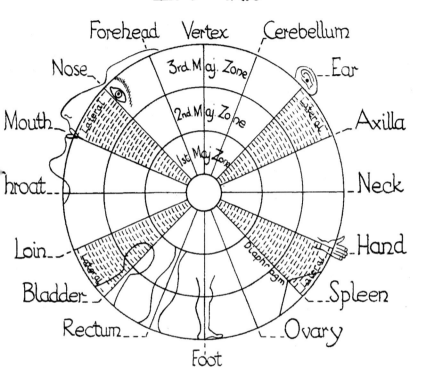

Forehead line ⎫
Ovary line ⎭ Sex line.

Mouth line ⎫
Hand line ⎭ Nutrition line.

Cerebellum line ⎫
Uterus line (rt.) ⎬ Sex line.
Rectum line (lt.) ⎭

Axilla line ⎫
Loin line ⎭ Endurance line.

Figure 5

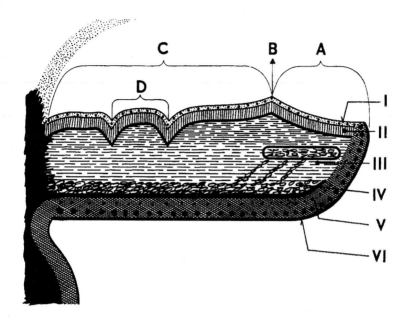

Schematic representation of the iris layers:

A Pupillary zone.
B Iris-wreath.
C Ciliary zone.
D Contraction rings.
 I Endothelial layer.
II Anterior marginal layer.
III Iris-stroma and vascular layer.
 IV Posterior marginal layer and dilatator layer.
 V Anterior pigment layer.
VI Posterior pigment layer = retinal layer.

95

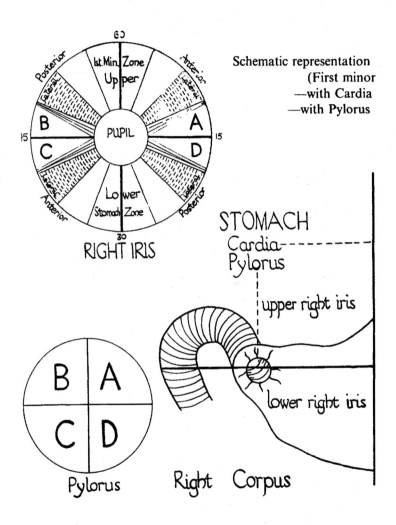

Schematic representation
(First minor
—with Cardia
—with Pylorus

Figure 6

of the Stomach zone
  zone).
= left iris.
= right iris.

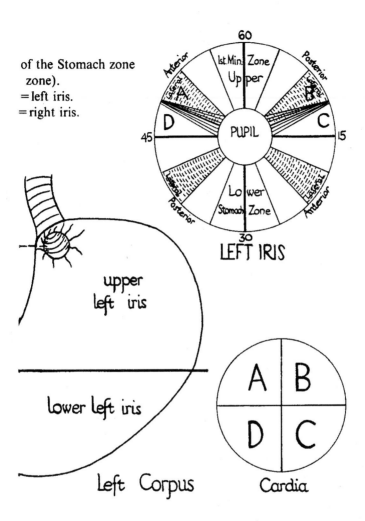

LEFT IRIS

upper
left iris

lower left iris

Left Corpus

Cardia

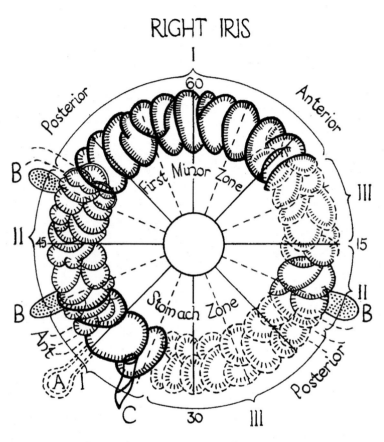

Schematic representation of the Intestinal zone (Second minor zone).

  I Ascending, transverse and descending colon.
 II Duodenum.
III Small intestine.
 IV Sigmoid flexure.
  V Rectum.

A Gall-bladder.
B Pancreas.
C Appendix.

Figure 7

LEFT IRIS

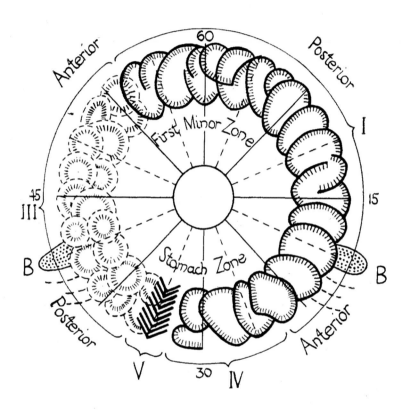

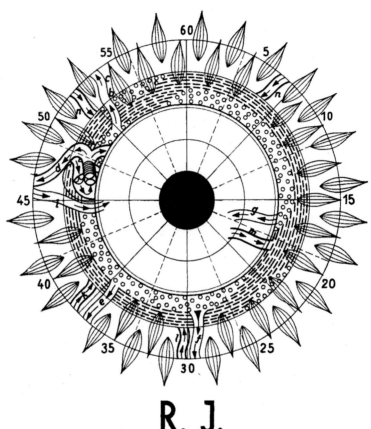

R. J.

Schematic representation of the Blood and Muscle zones
(Second major zone = third and fourth minor zones).

Right iris: Venous heart.   Left iris: Arterial heart.
o o o = arterial blood.   – – – = venous blood.

Figure 8

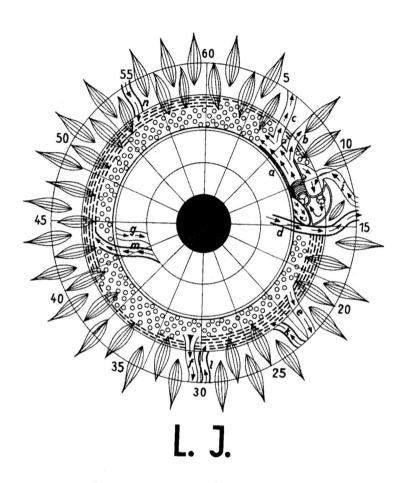

L. J.

(*a*) Aorta.   (*d*) Pulmonary artery.   (*g*) Gastric artery. Arterial supply
to arms (*b*), head (*c*), liver (*e*-rt.) and spleen (*e*-lt.), and legs (*f*).
(*i*) Pulmonary vein.   (*m*) Gastric vein.
Venous supply from liver (*k*-rt.) and spleen (*k*-lt.), head (*n*), and legs (*l*).

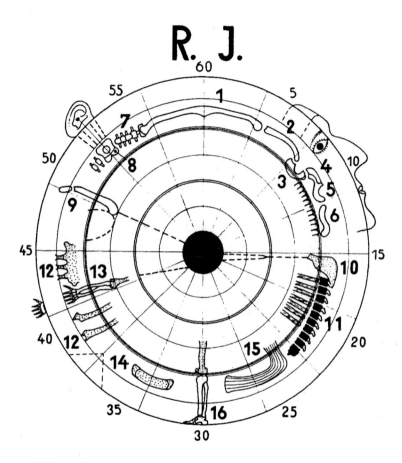

Schematic representation of the Bone zone (Fifth minor zone).

1 Cranial bone. 2 Frontal bone. 3 Orbit. 4 Nasal bone. 5 Upper jaw
and teeth. 6 Lower jaw and teeth. 7 Cervical vertebrae.

Figure 9

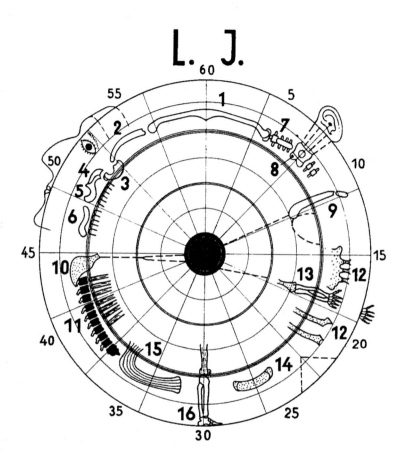

8 Ear. 9 Shoulder and clavicle. 10 Scapula. 11 Spine and ribs. 12 Sternum and ribs. 13 Hand and arm bones. 14 True pelvis. 15 Pelvic crests. 16 Foot and leg bones.

RIGHT IRIS

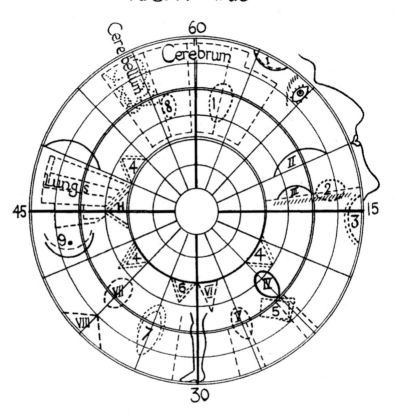

Schematic representation of the Second and Third major zones:

1 Pituitary. 2 Tonsils. 3 Thyroid. 4 Pancreas. 5 Prostate. 6 Supra-renal. 7 Ovary. 8 Pineal. 9 Mammary gland.

Figure 10

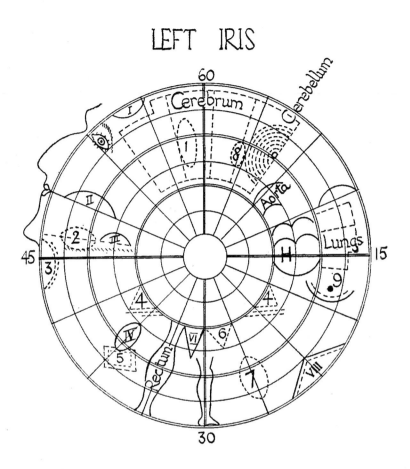

I Frontal sinus. II Palate. III Larynx. IV Urinary bladder. V Uterus.
VI Kidney. VII Gall-bladder. VIII Liver (rt. iris). Spleen (lt. iris).
H Heart.

RIGHT IRIS

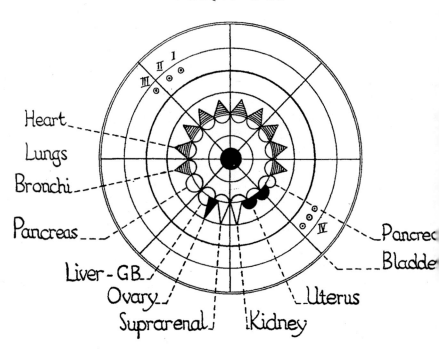

Heart
Lungs
Bronchi
Pancreas
Liver - G.B.
Ovary
Suprarenal
Kidney
Uterus
Pancrea
Bladde

Schematic representation of the Parasympathetic and Sympathetic Centres.

Parasympathetic nuclei: I Edinger-Westphal nucleus.
                         II Salivary nucleus.
                         III Vagal nucleus.
                         IV Sacral parasympathetic nuclei.

Figure 11

LEFT IRIS

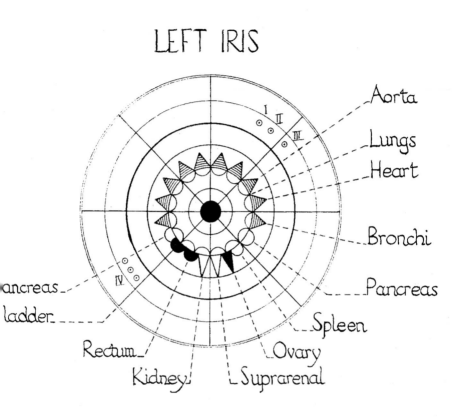

Sympathetic ganglia: ⩲ Superior, middle and inferior Cervical
        ganglia.
    ⌒ Coeliac and upper abdominal ganglia.
    ⬤ Lower abdominal ganglia.

Illustration 1

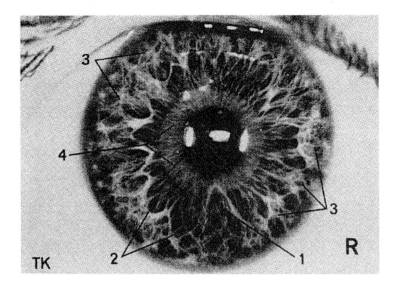

1 Contraction of the iris-wreath in the kidney area.
2 Dilatation of the iris-wreath in the area for ascending colon with indications of atrophy (Honeycomb signs).
3 Transversales = cobweb signs = adhesion signs.
4 Gastric hyperacidity (also see iris illus. 2).

Illustration 2

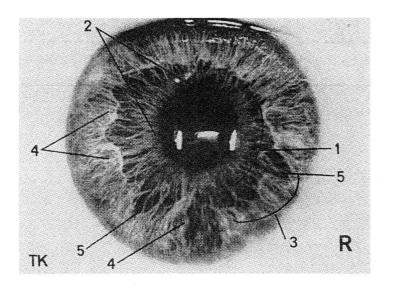

1 White inflammation signs in the outer part of the stomach ring.
2 Shadows from light reflex.
3 Dilatation of the iris-wreath from 17′–50′.
4 Contraction of the iris-wreath; in this case from a floating kidney (recognised by the arc-formation of the white lines traversing the leg area). Especially note the inflammation signs in this sector.
5 Atrophic signs = Honeycomb signs.

Illustration 3

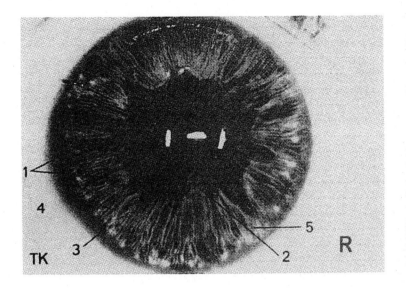

1 Contraction of the iris-wreath in the area for liver and lungs.
2 Contraction of the iris-wreath in the kidney area.
3 White flakes and clouds in the liver area.
4 Prominent vascular signs on the sclera adjacent to areas for liver and lungs.
5 Catarrh signs in the uterus area.
Otherwise, there is a considerable separation of the iris fibres with interspersed dark lines (the 'combed-hair' of Maubach). This, and the square-shaped iris-wreath indicate an incurable condition. Also note the black scurf-rim at 38′–48′ (also see iris illus. 7).

Illustration 4

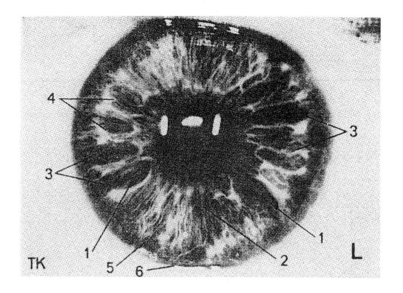

1 Lacuna in the pancreas area, with contraction of the iris-wreath.
2 Contraction of the iris-wreath in the areas for kidney and suprarenal gland.
3 Open lacunae.
4 Closed lacunae (see also iris illus. 5, 8, 9 and 11).
5 Inflammation- and haemorrhoid-signs in the area for rectum.
6 Transversal in the leg area after injury.

Illustration 5

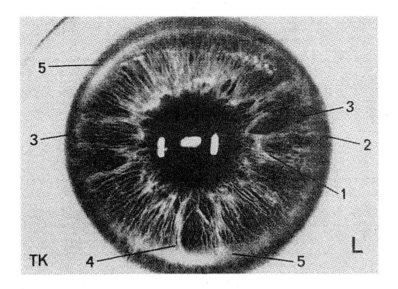

1 Thick white border around the iris-wreath with contraction in the heart area. (Calcification of the coronary vessels.)
2 White zigzag line extending out to the iris rim (cardiac neurosis).
3 Open lacunae.
4 Lacuna extending widthwise = stasis in the leg area (oedema).
5 Arcus senilis = senile ring.

Illustration 6

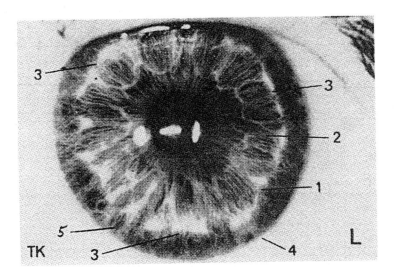

1 Transversal, running obliquely across the iris from the heart to the spleen area.
2 Dilatation of the iris-wreath below the heart area: Roemheld syndrome.
3 White clouds in the mucous membrane zone.
4 White wisp-signs = catarrh of the mucous membrane with elimination through the skin at 23′–27′.
5 Prominent signs of over-stimulation in the area for rectum. Note the transversales, half formed lacuna and the signs for loss of substance. The dark blood and muscle zone is also an indication of a general weakness.

Illustration 7

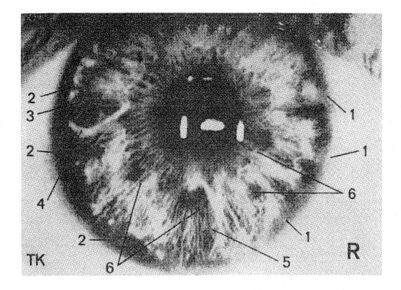

1 Large white wisp sign.
2 Black scurf-rim and flattening of the iris-rim adjacent to lung area at 47′–52′, with prominent blood vessels on the sclera.
3 Dissolution of the iris fibres as an indication of serious lung disease.
4 Thick white arc line as sign of inflammatory and exudative condition of the serous membranes.
5 Loosening of the iris fibres and contraction of the iris-wreath in the kidney area.
6 Large, almost black toxin-flecks.

Illustration 8

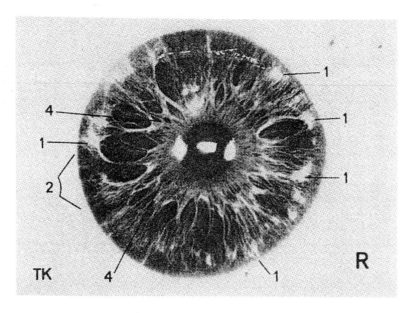

1 White flakes and wisps as indications of existing inflammation.

2 Darkening and arc-formation as signs of exudation. Transversales as signs of adhesions.

3 Several opened and closed lacunae in the respiratory organ areas and the kidney area.

4 Small black oblong signs inside the iris-wreath indicating ulcerous processes in the duodenum, with signs of encumbrance affecting the gall-bladder, liver and pancreas. The whole iris shows the general loosening of the iris fibres.

Illustration 9

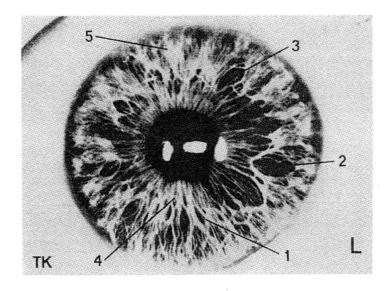

1 Suprarenal sign.
2 Heart lacuna, here displaced low because of the considerable dilatation of the iris-wreath (Roemheld).
3 Aortic lacuna lying too high.
4 Contraction of the iris-wreath as far as the pupillary margin in the kidney area. Also to be observed is the general overlaying throughout the iris with white clouds and flakes (Rheumatism).
5 Pituitary sign.

Illustration 10

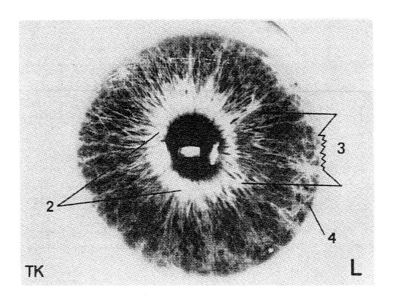

1 Oval pupil, and an almost unrecognisable first major zone, enables
  one to diagnose approaching death.
2 Thick white iris-wreath with radiating lines.
3 A thick white line running arc-shaped from 7′–20′ = calcification of
  the coronary vessels.
4 Transversal = cobweb sign in the pleural area. The separation of
  the iris fibres and the distribution of dark spots over the whole of the
  ciliary zone can also be seen.

Illustration 11

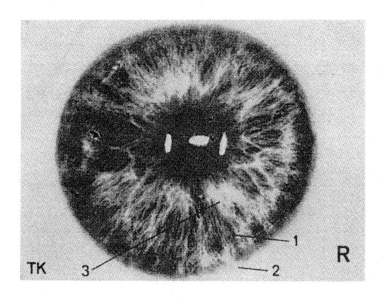

1 Uterine prolapse and displacement.
2 Sign for leucorrhoea.
3 Contraction of the iris-wreath in the areas for ovary and uterus. The Forehead-ovary line can be seen, as well as the two large heart-weakness signs at 42′–48′.

Illustration 12

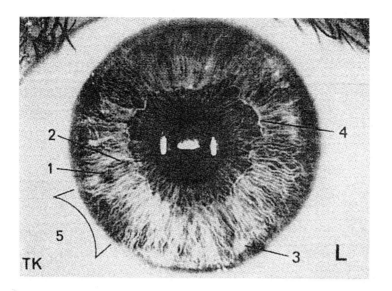

1 White lines running from the pupil to the outer iris rim. Black loss-of-substance signs with white clouds in the middle of the ciliary zone.
2 Displacement of the iris-wreath towards the pupil.
3 Sign for catarrh and swelling in the ovary area.
4 Dilatation of the iris-wreath in the areas for neck, shoulder and heart.
5 Transversales and angle-signs running from the outer rim inwards in the back area (injury). Also note the Axilla-loin line.

BIBLIOGRAPHY

ANGERER, Josef: *Handbuch der Augendiagnostik*, 1953.

BAUMHAUER, Karl: *Die Augendiagnose*, 1927.

FLINK, Frau Eva: *Zum 'Sehenlernen'*, EHK (Erfahrungsheilkunde), 1953.

Iriskorrespondenz, Jahrgänge, 1931–1937.

KRACK, Dr med N.: *Der Kopf an das Rückgrat nur angehängt*, EHK, 1961/5.

LANG, Walter, Dr med: *Die anatomischen und physiologischen Grundlagen der Augendiagnostik*, 1954.

MADAUS, Frau Magdalene: *Lehrbuch der Irisdiagnose*, 1926.

MAUBACH, A.: *Augendiagnostik*, 1952.

RAUBER-KOPSCH: *Anatomie III*, 1940.

ROSSDORF, Franz: *Einführung in die Augendiagnostik.*

SCHNABEL, Dr. Rudolph: *Ophthalmo-Symptomatologie*, 1952; *Iridoskopie*, 1959.

SCHULTE, Karl: *Encyklopädie der Irisdiagnostik*, 1938.

STRUCK-FLINK: *Irisdiagnose in der Praxis*, 1935.

THIEL, P. J.: *Der Krankheitsbefund aus den Augen*, 1921; *Die Augendiagnose*, 1929.

VIDA-DECK: *Klinische Prüfung der Organ- und Krankheitszeichen in der Iris*, 1954.